The
Book of Cuckoos

The Slim Girl's Book of Secrets

*Make today the last day
you ever worry about your
weight or appearance*

By Ali Campbell

Lowe & Campbell Publishing Ltd

This whole project could not have got off the ground never mind been completed without the help, love and support of many very special people.

Tim Lowe and Michael Neill – Simply thank you.
Alba Feely, Claire Horn and Janice Pitman – We couldn't have done it without you.

To my Mum and Dad – Thank you for everything, always. And to everyone else, too many people to mention you all here but I hope you know who you are. Whether you brought your inspiration or perspiration I will be forever grateful for your help.

Thank you all for being part of my life.

The Technical People –
Project Management: Martin Dowson and Ian Burgess
Design: Robert Gray
Printing and Binding: MPG Biddles

Finally, to you too, many thanks! I hope you enjoy what began as a daft idea in a coffee shop. May it help you to live the life you've always wanted and in ways you could only dream of... Ok, enough from me, best crack on!

Have fun, see you soon!
Ali x

The Slim Girl's Book of Secrets
Published by Lowe & Campbell Publishing Ltd,
Heather Lodge, Tower Road, Hindhead, Surrey GU26 6SU

British Library Cataloguing in Publication Data
A catalogue record for this book is available from the British Library

ISBN 978-0-9560805-0-9

Copyright © 2009 Ali Campbell and Lowe & Campbell Publishing Ltd

All rights reserved.

Apart from any use permitted under UK copyright law, this publication may only be reproduced, stored, or transmitted, in any form, or by any means, with prior permission in writing of the publishers or, in the case of reprographic production, in accordance with the terms of licences issued by the Copyright Licensing Agency.

Contents

Introduction 1
   How it Works for You   9
   Slim   10
   Fit   11
   Healthy   12
   Active   13
   Stylish   14

The Slim Girl's Key Secret CD 15
   Ready? Let's begin ...   16
   Your Journal   21

Slim 23

Slimming in Mind 51
   The Power of Intention   52

Fit 69
   Benefits of Exercise on your Energy Levels   71
   Benefits on Metabolism   73
   Benefits on your Body Shape and Body Confidence   76
   Health Benefits   78
   Weekly Plans and Progressions   103

Healthy 115

Active 159

Stylish 191
   Shape   202
   Conclusion   228
   In the Olympics of Life, We Could All Use a Coach   229

And Finally 233

Daily Do's 235

Introduction

As you sit and wonder how this book will be different, how this book will change your life when so many others have failed, I will let you in on a secret ... **This is not a diet book!**

That's right. This is not a diet book – this is a book about how to be slim and get the most out of your life.

In my time as a therapist, coach and mentor to some of the most famous, gifted, powerful and rich people on the planet I have learned to really live by my motto ... 'Never wonder what if ... '

Just go for it. Don't question what will happen once you have finished this book, just allow yourself to become absorbed in it and the rest is easy ... This book is written specifically to help you to become slimmer, fitter, and healthier and get more from your life. This is not a book about logic. You will not find any low fat recipes or calorie counting here, you'll not be weighing your food or counting your sin points. This is a book about the power of your mind, the power of your mind to make lasting changes in your body.

I'm guessing that one of the reasons you picked this way is because you're looking for an easy way to lose weight and get fit. Let's be honest, you chose this route because you have probably tried to do it the hard way already and you're curious to discover how the power of suggestion and the power of your mind really can overcome the urge for cheesecake and chocolate.

Well, you've come to the right place but you are going to have to be prepared to make changes more easily than you think.

INTRODUCTION

I am a hypnotherapist. What hypnotherapists do is to embed suggestions and commands in your subconscious mind using words so that you don't necessarily know why you do things differently, you just do. This book will not have you clucking like a chicken, I'm not a stage hypnotist but the effects you will notice can be just as dramatic. I have used all my skills here and have written this book to effortlessly change the way you think about and the relationship you have with food and with the rest of your life.

This is a special kind of book which just by reading it will help to redefine your relationship with food … It's not about starving yourself, it's not about sweating it out in the gym, and it's not about effort. It's about the little things that make a big difference. We're going to work together just as I have with thousands of people who, just like you have wanted to make big changes but weren't sure where to start. Just like you, they have tried and failed many times and, just like you will, they have achieved huge breakthroughs by simply following some of the suggestions you'll find here.

As I can't be there with you, I have filmed and recorded all of the techniques that you will need and I have even included a powerful CD for you to use daily, this will allow you to reshape the way you think about food. To ensure that **you** get the very best results, you have access to something that even my private clients don't have. You have the opportunity to benefit every day from the very latest psychological techniques to eliminate cravings and live life on your terms. Please do listen every day if you want to ensure the best results.

Another powerful difference is that I will personally guide you through all of the Do It *For* Yourself (DIFY) exercises. The important part of course is *'for'* yourself not *'by'* yourself. I am right here with you. They are all on the accompanying CD and in the same order as you'll find them here in the book. Each one has been recorded as if it were part of a real client session so you really are getting the same experience as one of my personal clients. I am not aware of this ever being done before, most audio CD's I have listened to sound a little staged. I didn't want to do this so what you have is just like the real thing, exactly what I do with someone just like you. I hope you enjoy the experience of working with me, I'm certainly looking forward to helping you.

You are holding in your hands the distilled learning and teaching I have gained from some of the very best therapists, coaches and trainers that I have had the pleasure to work with. I am combining the knowledge and skill I have gained as a Master Personal Trainer with those of Neuro Linguistic Programming, Hypnotherapy and Life Coaching so that I can help you to redefine your relationship with food once and for all.

That's a potent mix. It's a formula that I first tried and tested in Scotland, probably the most cynical and according to the *Scottish Sunday Mail*, also the second fattest country in the world behind the USA. I have now taken these techniques around the world and across many cultures and one thing is constant – This way works!

INTRODUCTION

You are about to experience an amazing journey of self-discovery and change for the better.

I know that by now you will be curious to know where we're going to start. Well, we're going to start by letting go of limiting beliefs, by letting go of that tried and failed attitude. I guess you've tried diets before and they didn't work for you, or they worked for a little while then you put all the weight, and more, back on. You have made the right move. You can give up on diets for good. Remember this is not a diet book and you're not alone. Let's have a look at some scientific fact for a second. The following extract is from a *Medicare* report published in '*American Psychologist*'

> ### Medicare's Search for Effective Obesity Treatments
> *Diets Are Not the Answer*
>
> The prevalence of obesity and its associated health problems have increased sharply in the past 2 decades. New revisions to Medicare policy will allow funding for obesity treatments of proven efficacy. The authors review studies of the long-term outcomes of calorie-restricting diets to assess whether dieting is an effective treatment for obesity.
>
> These studies show that one third to two thirds of dieters regain **more** weight than they lost on their diets, and these studies likely underestimate the extent to which dieting is counterproductive because of several methodological problems, all of which bias the studies toward showing successful weight loss maintenance. In addition, the studies do not provide consistent evidence that dieting results in significant health improvements, regardless of weight change. **In sum, there is little support for the notion that diets lead to lasting weight loss or health benefits**.
>
> (*American Psychologist*, April 2007, Vol. 62, No. 3)

What does that tell us? It tells us that it's not your fault! I cannot stress that enough, it's not your fault! You tried it, it didn't work for you and it's time to move on. I'm sure in many areas of your life you have tried something, it's not worked out and you've moved on without a second thought. So why do you beat yourself up about dieting and failing? The answer here is simple, in society we are conditioned to crave being thin ... the media is full of pictures of stick thin airbrushed models.

My definition of model is simple 'like the real thing only smaller'. We crave being thin and are made to feel bad when the solution we are force-fed doesn't work. It's not your fault. The diet industry has conditioned you to feel bad when their product fails.

It must be one of the few industries where when their product fails they make out that it's your fault ... Now, in this book I choose my words carefully. Did you notice I used diet 'industry' and 'product'? That's quite deliberate. The diet industry is worth billions of pounds every year and you are the one losing pounds but only into their coffers.

I'm so glad you've seen the light at last and recognise that being slim is about a state of mind rather than counting calories.

I'm looking forward to helping you to become slimmer, fitter, and healthier as well as enjoying being more active in the rest of your life. The first thing you need to do before we start is to begin to let go of the idea that you are overweight. We all have an idea in our minds of who we are and what we look like. This is one of the

INTRODUCTION

main reasons why our weight may fluctuate but it almost always returns to the mental image we have of ourselves. Before we change the way others see you, it's time to change the way you see yourself. Let's have a look at the way you can be once you absolutely know how.

I'd like you to take a moment and close your eyes ... Ok, you're right that won't work, on second thoughts, read the next bit then close your eyes. I'd like you to close your eyes and make a picture of yourself. We're not going to change anything just yet; I'm going to make you wait a little longer to get to the juicy stuff. Just close your eyes and notice the image you have of yourself. Is it anything like you actually look? If it's an overweight you, imagine yourself slim and fit and healthy.

Please don't read on yet, stop and imagine yourself slim and fit and healthy ... Some people really struggle to do this – they can make a picture of a slim fit and healthy person maybe that's you? But they can't put their face on it. Try it just now. Is that you? Now float yourself into that picture so that you see yourself through your own eyes, notice what it's like to see through the eyes of a slim person, a slim you. You may not be able to make a picture of the slim you with your face but you will be able to make a picture of a slim body and then float into it.

Float into it and then run the movie that you see from your ideal eyes, take yourself through an ideal day. Notice how people react to the slimmer you, notice how you think and feel. Then find the best part about being that person. What is it that you enjoy most about spending time in the ideal you? What do you do then that you can't do now? Just run the movie forward again now and really enjoy connecting with the real you.

Is it that you look great and people compliment you?

Is it that you're no longer arguing with yourself about food or have stopped worrying about what people think?

How does the world react differently to you? I had a client once who rightly said that the weird thing about gaining weight was that the bigger she got, the less visible she became. She's right and I'm sure you've noticed that too. The more weight you gain the less people notice you. Service isn't as good in restaurants, heads no longer turn when you walk into a room and I know you know how bad those stick thin young shop assistants can make you feel when you ask for a bigger size. Imagine all that changing. Imagine slipping into those skinny jeans again or make a picture of whatever your measure of success will be.

Please, please, please, when we're talking about how to measure your success, please (have I stressed that enough?) do not use scales! Not for a while anyway.

Just wait 'til you feel your waistband looser for the first time or the first time someone compliments you on looking great. That'll feel better and give you more motivation than scales ever could.

Perhaps I'll just explain a little about how this book works as it's a bit different to others. Ok it's a lot different. If you're wondering when we're going to get started,

INTRODUCTION

we already have ... As you read and as you enjoy the stories and techniques your subconscious will take in my suggestions, even if you don't consciously notice them you will be affected by these words just the same.

I guess I should give you the option though. If you don't want to be affected by my words and powerful psychological techniques and therefore stay as you are then you'd better put the book down and go make a cup of tea now!

How it Works for You

Ok – great, so I'll assume that if you're still with me then you're ready to make a difference to your life and of course your waistline.

For ease, this book is split into 5 sections

Slim
Fit
Healthy
Active
Stylish

I have chosen these words as they are the ones most commonly used by my clients when they want to change the way they are and the quality of life they enjoy.

Whilst at first glance these terms might appear similar let me explain the difference, as you'll understand them here.

Slim

Slim may be a physical appearance but it's more a state of mind. In this section we're going to dispel the myths of dieting and train you to think and act like a thin person. You'll be well aware that 'will power' doesn't work; you've tried that already. Here you'll understand the psychological differences that really change your relationship with food. The best bit of all is that will power is not required. This is not a book on logic; logically you know what you should be eating already. You probably know the calorific value of foods better than many a nutritionalist. That's not the point. The difference between success and failure is in doing it and to keep doing it and that's where logic often fails. Emotions are not logical nor is your relationship with food. And that's why we do it differently here.

You'll be able to change the way you think about food and enjoy that relationship on your terms.

It's time to dump logical diets and use your emotions for good.

In this section we are going to set about putting right the bad habits that diets have conditioned you with and heal the scars that constantly beating yourself up have left. We are going to do some work, just as I do with my private clients to quickly put you back on track. You are one of my clients now and I'm going to take care of you.

INTRODUCTION

The author and coach Maria Nemeth once shared the following analogy for what it's like when she meets with a new client for the first time:

"Imagine a person standing in front of you complaining they can't walk properly because of a sore foot. As they're calling your attention towards their foot, you can't help noticing that they're holding a gun directly above it, pointing straight down. Next, you notice they have a severe twitch every couple of minutes, and that every time they twitch the gun goes off, sending another bullet directly into the foot.

No matter how enthusiastic and motivated they are to begin moving forward, it would be a waste of time to work on getting anywhere or even on healing their wounded foot until you did something about the gun and the twitch."

Similarly, when we begin to work together we're going to start by laying the foundations, putting things right and making sure you're not shooting yourself in the foot.

Fit

This section will again be a little different from most exercise 'wisdom' you've come across. The physiology and exercise theory is sound but the delivery is a little different. What you'll find here is designed to be the most efficient way to use your time and get the maximum return for your effort. Did I mention I used to run competitively and be a Master Personal Trainer? Again, the difference lies not in whether the techniques are backed by the latest cutting edge biomechanical theory, or which celebrity is endorsing the program, the difference is in whether you actually do it or not.

The exercises you will be guided through by Alba (she is my Personal Trainer) are designed to give you the most return for each bead of sweat you invest. We have chosen them specifically because they will give you the greatest benefit for the least effort. Please don't get me wrong if you want to do more I will back you all the way but this doesn't have to be about hard training and sweating in the gym. These exercises can be done at home using only a couple of things you'll have lying around. We have made this as easy as possible for you. Many people have lost a lot of weight using these techniques without doing any structured exercise at all. However, if you want to get the best results and fast, then a few minutes per day will make all the difference.

Healthy

How will you know when you feel healthy? It's one of those terms that get trotted out all the time but what does it mean to you? Will it be when you have more energy? Will it be when you catch a glimpse of your reflection and really like what you see? Or will it be when you have a sense of calm and ease in your daily life. In my book health is different from fitness. You can be fit but not healthy. 'Health' is about balance and a sense of well-being. It's not about material stuff, it's

INTRODUCTION

about being happy ... Imagine being slim, fit AND happy. I know it all seems too good to be true but you have to be prepared to do things differently. The definition of insanity could be 'doing the same thing over and over and expecting a different result'. It's time to stop repeating old habits and feel happy and healthy in yourself for a change.

Active

Ok so you're slim, you're fit, you're happy and you're healthy ... What are you going to do next? This is the section where you make some big plans and your dreams come true. Now that you have no reason not to, what would you really love to do? We will set some goals but as you may have guessed already, this won't be in the usual way. You can use some of the techniques here to help you earn more money, have more quality time with your loved ones or to get more from your career. I'm not content with you just being slim I want to help you to love your life and live to your full potential.

While I hope you will get something from every exercise in this book I know from experience that you will have particular favourites. Simply turn down the corner of the pages that you enjoy most and you'll be able to quickly find them again ... In the active section we will combine your favourite parts and apply them and others to getting the most out of your future. Ok, I hope all that made sense, if it hasn't yet I'm sure it will once we get going.

Stylish

To top it all off I have included a style section. Now I'll confess that I know little or nothing about this subject (I don't think men are supposed to) but you don't have to be an expert to be able to find one. So, just as I have done with the fitness section, I went out and found you someone who really does know their stuff then persuaded them to share their trade secrets with me so that I can share them with you. Shhh … don't tell anyone.

What you will find here is the combined wisdom of our secret stylist in the industry and of course my take on the psychology behind it.

If you're like me and find that you normally pick the same colours and styles then the colour analysis tool kit will almost certainly have you shopping in a whole new way in future. Colour is a huge factor in how we look and feel, so I have included a simple colour analysis kit so that you can find your natural skin tone and shop like the stylists.

You will also be able to analyse your own face shape and be guided as to which hair style is perfect for you, identify your body shape and learn some of the professional secrets to choosing the right cut and fabric to show off and enhance your natural assets. What could be better than being slim, fit, healthy, active and doing so with a sense of flair and style?

The Slim Girl's Key Secret CD

The audio CD that you have in your box is a recording of the powerful life-changing techniques that I have used countless times to help reprogram the habits and behaviours of my personal clients.

This is a blended mix of the latest psychological techniques that I have refined and tailored so that you will lose weight effortlessly and without dieting.

It is very powerful. Please do not use it when you are driving, operating machinery or are in any way responsible for the wellbeing of others. Please only listen to it when you can safely relax completely and just allow the sounds to wash over you. It works and is a key part of this weight loss package. For best results use it every day. I would suggest that you should use it in the morning. This is for 2 reasons: Firstly it will set you up by conditioning your attitude to food for the day ahead like never before and secondly, as it is designed to leave you feeling fully refreshed and energised, you might find it difficult to get to sleep if you listen to it last thing at night.

Ready? Let's begin ...

I have often thought that the hardest step on any journey is the first one. My athletics coach used to always say that the toughest step in training was the first one out of the front door. I have to say that, while I understood his point, the last few steps of a race definitely hurt more ... None of that for you though, and I'd like to begin by congratulating you on making it this far.

THE SLIM GIRL'S KEY SECRET CD

You've taken the hardest step and embarked on a journey of change. This book is very different from others you'll have read and instead of talking about what you will be going without (that's what diets do) here we'll be talking about what you are gaining and moving towards. As this is the first week, I'll be both easy and hard on you to begin with. It's simple but not easy: simple in that you don't really have to do much this week, the suggested exercise is very light and the Do It *For* Yourself parts are simple. However, that's not to say they are easy. I want to radically change the way you think about yourself and your relationship with food. We're going to challenge some of your current beliefs and change the way you think for good. If you don't understand straight away, don't worry, why should you? You've never done it this way before. If you feel confused at any point, just go back and read it again. I want you to think of confusion as a good thing, confusion is a step on the path to understanding. If you think about anything new that you have learned in the past I'm sure, at some point, it felt a little strange and confusing before you fully understood it and it became second nature to you.

In the work I have done on weight loss with literally thousands of people around the world a few fundamentals hold true …

1 You probably think about food a disproportionate amount of the time. Even if it's thinking 'I don't want

that' or 'I shouldn't have that' it's still thinking about food. It's ok we're going to change that.
2 You quite possibly eat very quickly. Let's change that too.
3 You probably feel a sense of loss if you go without or deprive yourself of some 'treat' that you think you'd really enjoy.
4 And you definitely wish that if only there was a magic answer then you would do whatever it took to get that pill or potion that would change your life.

I'm going to ask you to do things differently, but you know that (after all you've tried the other ways and that's why you're reading this now).

I'm not a magician but you do have a magic formula in your hands right now ... I can't stress this enough. Give this program and yourself an honest chance and in 5 weeks from now you will be looking back at the old you and wondering why you didn't do it sooner. 5 weeks is not a long time ...

Take a moment to think what you were doing 5 weeks ago, can you even remember? I'm sure it doesn't feel that long at all. As I write this, it's the end of January and Christmas was only 5 weeks ago. Frankly, it feels like 5 minutes. In our busy lives, time passes so quickly we hardly even notice. Over the next weeks, you have the chance to make a lifetime of difference Let's begin with our first exercise ... Once you have read the DIFY Exercise, take a few moments to do it and notice how it feels.

THE SLIM GIRL'S KEY SECRET CD

Remember all the DIFY exercises are on CD for you. Just follow the track listing shown.

1 – DIFY – Timeline

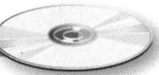

In a moment I'd like you to close your eyes ... (not yet though) and if you would like some extra guidance you will find me talking you through this and all the DIFY exercises on the audio CD in your Box of Secrets. I should point out that most of the exercises here will be with your eyes closed. This is simply because with your eyes closed you can make better pictures.

I'd like you to take a moment and just close your eyes and point in the direction of the future. Most people have a sense of which way the future is, with the opposite direction being their past.

Once you have a sense of the direction of your future I'd like you to imagine a line running away from you through time, off into the distance. This is your time line and we'll be returning to it later. The first thing I'd like you to do is to get a sense of scale. How far in the future is tomorrow? You'll just get a sense of what feels right for you. How far ahead is next week, next month, next year? Make a little mental note in your mind. Now, float yourself up over your time-line and take yourself to a place some time from now, when you are exactly the way you'd love to be. Slim, Fit, Healthy and Active. What do you notice about yourself that you like most? Is it the way you walk? The way you have more energy? The sense of ease? Or is it simply the way you can wear whatever you want? Notice where you are on your timeline and make another little mental mark. Now, in your head I'd like you to turn around to face back towards now and notice how far you have come. You might even have a sense of the weeks or months that separate the ideal you from where you started. You'll also notice how relatively short that time is and how effortless the transition was. It's always easier to look back than forward but from this place of achievement you can get a sense of perspective. Five weeks may sound like a long time today, perhaps not quick enough or a little daunting. But go to the end of the journey and look back and it always feels much easier.

Have you ever noticed that when you go on holiday the journey home always feels shorter than going? That's because, on the way out you don't know what to expect so you set an expectation that feels 'about right'. It's almost always worse than the reality. Whereas, on the return journey, you know what to expect and frame it accordingly.

Go to the point on your time line where you've achieved your goal and, as you look back, really allow yourself to notice how easy it has been. Are you surprised? Get a feel for the journey in your head and then notice where you 'feel' your significant way markers are. Your initial milestone, then the part where you know for sure that you are changing for good and then the final 'ideal' you.

You don't need to be precise or logical just go to where 'feels about right' to you. Maybe it's the first time you notice your clothes feel looser or the first compliment you're paid on your new look. Then, notice other significant steps on the journey you are taking to a slimmer, fitter, happier and more active you.

For now, just get a feel for where they are on your timeline and you will begin to get a sense of when it feels like you will achieve your initial goal, whatever that may be for you. I say initial goal, because it's my hope that this book will not just help you to lose weight and feel great, it will give you a whole new way of looking at your life and a bunch of techniques that you can use long after you have achieved your ideal weight.

When you have done that, you can open your eyes and note down your way markers in your journal. You'll enjoy ticking these off as we move forward and you might surprise yourself at just how accurate you are.

Your Journal

You will notice that you have a journal section for each day of the first 5 weeks we'll spend together. You can use this to record anything you like (or dislike) about your day. It can range from the profound to the ridiculous; the journal is here for you for 2 reasons.

- Firstly, it's really useful to keep track of any journey and this one is no different. Record your successes, the exercises that you liked, the insights you have gained and the progress you are making.
- The second reason for the journal is that this book is not about reading, it's about doing.

I once had a client, although I'm sure they're not alone, who told me they regularly sat down with a self help book, read it from cover to cover (as if it was a novel) but didn't ever consider doing any of the things it suggested. Now that to me seems a little silly. Why put in all the effort of reading the book if you're not actually going to DO it? I would love this book to become your companion, your friend and your secret diary for the next 5 weeks. It's you and me and together we're going to get you back on track and losing weight easily.

Slim

While this Box of Secrets is definitely about being slim, that's only one part of it. So, as you read on I'd like you to start by being a bit kinder to yourself and begin by stopping beating yourself up for not being perfect. Stop comparing yourself to everyone else and enjoy being you. You are amazing, kind, loving, giving, curious and full of the wonderful things that make you, you. The fastest way to make yourself feel bad is to compare your inside to someone else's outside. Please stop, it's not good for you.

While I'm on the subject, I'd like to ask a favour of you? Please, for now don't tell anyone we're working together … I want this to be your special time and your special journey. Our little secret! Your friends and family will notice soon enough when they're seeing a lot less of you. Let me explain why I ask this, it's certainly not that I'm ashamed of our relationship here.

I have learned over the years that self assembled support groups tend not to work very well. People tend to be 'supportive' only within the boundaries of their own limitations and expectations. I'm sure you've been in situations where you have started out on a diet or fitness kick or New Year resolution with a friend. You have right? So, how did it go? Let me take a guess … either, you were doing well, then the other person couldn't make it for some reason? Or they didn't stick to the diet that week? Or had a 'very good reason' why they couldn't join you? If this happened, then one of 3 things almost inevitably also happened.

1 You secretly felt a sense of relief that you hadn't been the first one to break and showed solidarity with your friend by falling by the wayside too.

2 You carried on but your friend became progressively less supportive until you stopped as you didn't want to make them feel bad or you began to feel like you didn't fit in anymore.

3 You went into it together with the same 'stated desire' but neither of you really had the belief that change was possible and so you 'encouraged' each other that it was too hard and you'd best just stay the same.

It's true of many group situations. While groups can bond and be supportive, just as often they don't. I remember early on in my career being invited to speak to a group of agoraphobics (fear of the outdoors or busy places). Now, whichever genius had organised this had booked a venue right in the middle of the city at 9.30am. Handy for me, but the people who were attending had to travel considerable distances on busy trains or in heavy traffic just to get there. Genius! I think not ... If the people weren't anxious enough already, they certainly were by the time they arrived!

What happened next was even more remarkable. The group were encouraged to speak about their condition and their experiences and, one by one, they each took turns at outdoing each other about just how bad their lives were and what they weren't able to do. It was the most bizarre thing ever. Just by being there they had proved that they could go out and travel but by doing the group session they painstakingly reinforced their condition and their attachment to it ... The session was well intentioned but totally bonkers!

I have seen something similar in diet groups. The strange thing in this situation is that, although you might not realise it, you actually have a vested interest in the other person failing. After all, if they succeed and you don't, what does that say about you? I'm not saying that people would deliberately sabotage someone else's efforts at losing weight but the person who is less committed (and someone always is) certainly has a vested interest in maintaining the status quo.

This probably sounds counter intuitive to all the diet clubs and groups who advocate camaraderie and team work. That may be the mission statement but the underlying fact of *motivation through guilt* is not a healthy way to achieve any goal. I know you'll know someone (it might even be you) who has eaten all the wrong things all week then starved themselves the day before the dreaded weigh-in so that they don't feel the public shame of standing on the scales and hearing the words 'this week ... 'no change', or worse, 'a gain'!

In my book, this is no way to motivate anyone to do anything. It's a bit like when you were at school and the teacher shamed you into remembering your gym kit by making those who'd forgotten it take PE in their pants. You might do it but very grudgingly and only for as long as you really have to. You'll try to stick with your diet until either you break or your 'diet buddy' breaks and lets you off the hook.

You might think I'm being a bit harsh but I've heard it so many times from so many people that I know it's true …

So I'd like you to keep what we're doing as our little secret. You have something very special in your hands. It's a new way of thinking, a new way of being and, as this is my first book, it's something that not many people have yet. I'm honoured to have the chance to share the secrets and tips that have helped my private clients to live the lives of their dreams with you. All I ask is that you do what I suggest and keep it to yourself for now. Once you have dropped a couple of dress sizes, notches on your belt (or whatever your particular goal is) I'd love you to shout from the roof tops how you did it, but for now, let's keep this between you and me.

This is not a logical book, you will be asked to do things that you have never done before and that might at first seem a little odd or have nothing to do with weight loss. Trust me they do!

What you will not find is counting calories, counting sin points, counting the minutes 'til your next meal, weighing out your ingredients, cutting out food groups or multiplying the amount of fat by 9 then dividing by the number you first thought of … Argh! That's all much too much like hard work. And it often doesn't work.

So, what's the secret of losing weight and keeping it off? It's actually surprisingly simple: the real key to losing weight and keeping it off is to listen to your body in a state where you are free from the emotional attachment to food.

If you have a bad food day, it's not the end of the world. Just get back on track tomorrow. You are not perfect and you have to live so cut yourself some slack and get on with it. I'd like you to think about your program as a bank account. Every time you do well it's like putting money in the weight loss bank. Every time you fall off the wagon, or over indulge, it's like making a withdrawal. The key is not to go bankrupt!

Before we get on to the really cool stuff there are a few fundamentals to get right. The techniques that follow are potent yet simple. You may have seen some of them elsewhere and that's because they are the ones that work. I am not claiming to have reinvented the wheel here. What I have done is bring together the most potent change techniques in one place and in a way that you cannot help but change easily as you read on. If you have seen some of these before, please do take note anyway, it's the order and the way that they are presented here that makes the difference. Please do not skip ahead. I'm not there with you so I need to rely on you reading my words, they're all specifically chosen here to help you. I know that you will be keen to get to the juicy bits but it's time to do things differently and take a little time to overcome your emotions and make a difference.

You may not think that you are emotionally attached to food, but it's almost certain you are. Phrases like 'comfort eating' or 'feel good food' have crept into our vocabulary. It feels like they've always been there. But they haven't. Why would food give you comfort? Why would sugar, salt, fat and wheat give you comfort? Surely comfort should be found in other things? I had a particularly overweight client once who sought comfort in all the 'wrong' things. She even sabotaged all the good and hard work she was putting in at the gym by seeking comfort in food.

I'm going back a few years now but at the time I was working with this lady as her personal trainer and she had just done a fantastic session in the gym with me. She really worked hard and I remember congratulating her on burning lots of calories and feeling so pleased with myself that I had got her to a point where she was actually enjoying our exercise sessions.

I really thought she had turned a corner. You see, she was successful in all the other areas of her life. She had a beautiful flat in a great part of town, was director of a company that was doing well and I really envied her little sports car. Her aspiration, she said, was to look as if she 'should' be driving it. In other words, she wanted to look like the kind of person who would pose around town in a little red soft top.

It was that car, however, that was to be her downfall that night. After a brilliant session with her in the gym, I packed up and was heading home. On my journey I noticed that same little red sports car parked on the street and my heart sank! After all our hard work and all my pep talks and all her affirmations and goals and dreams, the car was parked outside … the chip shop. I remember feeling gutted, as much for me as for her. I felt like I had failed her in some way, like I hadn't been motivational enough. Like I hadn't helped her to believe …

Then I remember feeling angry because she was letting herself down and me for that matter. I had put so much effort into her training plan and her nutritional plan and her life plan and here she was in the takeaway undoing all of the hard work we had both put in. WHY?

I guess the answer was simple really. It wasn't that she didn't appreciate me (believe me, we personal trainers take it very 'personally' when clients sabotage themselves). It wasn't that she didn't want the outcome and didn't want to flash around in that convertible. It was simply that she had a really strong emotional attachment to food and that particular night she was treating herself because she had done so well ... Argh!

Not her fault and not yours either. We are conditioned to be emotionally attached to food. It's the way we are brought up and it's the way society shapes us – literally! When we're young and we're good we get a treat! Tidy your room and you'll get a treat; finish your homework and you'll get a sweet, do well in your exams and we'll go out for a nice meal to celebrate. Or, we seek out comfort in food. You're not well, so have something nice to make you feel better; you're feeling down, have something nice to cheer yourself up. It's food, food, food. Clear your plate and you'll get a lolly ... And that's another thing, how many of you are fully paid up members of the plate clearer club?

Leave food on your plate

If you don't finish everything on your plate it's a waste right? Wrong! If you don't eat it, it goes in the bin. If you do eat it, it goes down the loo. The only difference is that, with the second option, some of it sticks to 'your waistline'. It's a waste as soon as you cook more than you need. It doesn't matter whether it goes past you or through you, it's heading in the same direction. Make no mistake, either way it's wasted.

If you clear your plate – it's your waist

Studies have shown that, as a nation, we were healthiest in Britain during the Second World War. Ok, that's not strictly true, people suffered in many other ways but our diets were the healthiest they've ever been during the rationing of wartime.

Many people were better fed during wartime food rationing than either before or after the war years. Infant mortality rates declined and the average age at which people died from natural causes increased.

The wartime food shortages forced people to adopt new eating patterns. Most people ate less meat, fat, eggs and sugar than they had eaten before. You were only allowed one egg and 3 rashers of bacon a week but Britons were never healthier than when we lived on wartime rations.

Today, almost a quarter of all adults in the UK are obese.

Even more horrifying, a quarter of all British toddlers are already overweight.

Our diet contains too much fat, sugar and salt – and it's putting us at greater risk of diabetes, heart disease, cancer, stroke and even Alzheimer's.

THE SLIM GIRL'S BOOK OF SECRETS

Under rationing, every adult was allowed 8oz (230g) of sugar a week. On average we have twice that now.

Just one bowl of a typical breakfast cereal, a serving of baked beans with lunch and a Jaffa Cake would take you over your World War II sugar ration without so much as a sprinkling of the white stuff.

As well as affecting dental health, excess sugar consumption has been linked to weight gain, diabetes and, by some experts, even to cancer.

When the British *Daily Mail* conducted an experiment asking a modern family to live on wartime rationing, the results were startling.

The first thing I noticed was how little food we were wasting. Because we all snack throughout the day, no one is hungry at meal times and I frequently throw good food in the bin. But because supplies were limited, I had to serve smaller portions, I also had more energy, and our digestive systems seemed to benefit – we've both become wonderfully regular in our trips to 'the loo'.

But I think the real transformation was in the children: they slept better, had more energy and weren't as "hyper"; there was markedly less fighting and whingeing but now that we've gone back to our old food, the tantrums and general irritability levels have started to rise.

Now I'm not suggesting that we go back to such draconian measures. After all, that was a very long time ago and affected a different generation right? Well that's where you're wrong. I'm sure you, like me, were told when we were growing up that leaving food was a waste. You might have already passed that on to your own children. Your parents may even have been like mine and wrapped and saved every possible scrap of left over food to be used in some casserole, soup or for sandwiches the next day. Food was thought of as precious and shouldn't be wasted. It wasn't really that precious and it certainly wasn't as scarce as it had been but that mental programming carried over from the war generation into my parents and, I'm sure, into yours too.

Food was precious and should not be wasted. My Mum has an extensive list of recipes you simply cannot cook from scratch; they all involve leftovers of some kind. I think a lot of our favourite dishes are based on using up ingredients so they don't go to waste. We have a mental programme giving us the message that food is scarce and precious and must not be wasted. If it's on my plate, it must be eaten and she who has food is lucky, abundant, rich or fortunate, or frugal, thrifty and therefore a good person. How silly is that? If we don't throw away a small bit of food or eat more than we need, it means all of those things, we are a good person, we have good values … hmmm.

When that way of thinking is dropped into a world where food could not be more plentiful or cheap, is it any wonder that we eat too much? Can you see how this works now? We are programmed to value and covet food yet food could not be more plentiful.

As a society we are obsessed with food. And yet food has never ever been more readily available or convenient. Is it any wonder that when you mix the desire to have food with such abundance, things go a little mad? Add to that all the emotional stuff around comfort food and you can quickly see how it all went wrong ... I want you to stop now and take stock of your attitude and relationship with food. Please be very honest with yourself here.

Just answer the following questions and complete the statements to get an idea of how you really think about it. Don't think about your answers just go with the first thing that comes to mind. A bit like playing a word association game.

2 | DIFY – Attitude to food, word association game.

1. Food is ...
2. The best thing about food is ...
3. I love food because ...
4. Food makes me feel ...
5. I have a ... relationship with food
6. I keep my relationship this way because ...
7. The worst thing about it being this way is ...
8. The thing I'd like to change most is ...
9. I've not changed it yet because ...
10. Is that last answer a 'fact' a 'possible fact' or an 'assumption'?
11. If it's a fact, how do you know that for sure?
12. If it's a possible fact – what might be the opposite, which might also be true?

If it's an assumption – what might really be true if only you were brave enough to admit it now?

Ok, so we've done a bit of uncovering the real attitude you have to food. That's the 'why you eat' part. Now go back through your list and notice what some of the thoughts might have been around your answers. Log what you find in your journal.

Know when to eat?

Now it's time to have a think about when we eat. You see again we are all programmed and conditioned to eat at certain times. Morning coffee, breakfast time, elevenses, lunchtime, afternoon tea, (I'm sounding like a hobbit), dinnertime, teatime and then supper. Now I'm sure, as you read this, you are thinking "Yes, but I don't have all of those". I'm sure that's true but that doesn't include snacks and drinks. A quick snack and a latté can have as many calories as half the daily War Time diet. I am a fully paid up member of the Starbucks fan club but did you know that a venti white chocolate double whip mocha and a blueberry muffin contains 1067 calories? I'm guessing not. And a normal grande latté and muffin racks up 672 calories. Go skinny and leave the muffin, it really does make quite a difference. A grande skinny latté has only 131 calories. Not a bad saving for virtually no difference in taste.

Ok, so we've gone skinny but I'll bet you still eat when you think you're supposed to? Who is it that dictates you should eat at certain times? I'm not sure either because, unless you live in an institution and are forced to conform, I would suggest that a far healthier strategy would be to eat when you're hungry …

It just sounds more sensible to me. Your body is equipped with an early warning signal to let you know that it needs some food and I, for one, would suggest that you listen to it. Now here's a question …

3 | DIFY – Are you feeling hungry? – Really?

When was the last time you felt hungry? I know the quick answer is probably 'this morning' or 'at lunch time' or 'I'm always hungry' but let me ask you 'is that a physical hunger or an emotional hunger?'

I bet you can catch yourself saying 'I'm hungry' or 'I feel like a …' when what you actually mean is 'I have an emotional need for food'.

True hunger is a feeling in your stomach. A feeling, not a craving or an urge or a habit. Think about the question again, when was the last time you felt hungry?

I last felt physically hungry ………………………………

I knew it was genuine hunger because ……………………

The time before that was ……..………………………….

We can feel like we need food for a number of reasons but let me share some of the common ones with you here … I'd like you to think about 'you' as you read through the next section. If any of these strike a chord just make a mental note; 'Yip, that's definitely me sometimes'.

- **Am I tired?** – In our busy lives we all get tired, burning the candle at both ends trying to juggle so many things and get everything done. Make sure you are not depleting your energy and trying to get it from food alone.

We need 7–8 hours sleep per night to ensure our body's health and well-being. Some people can function well on less, but on average increasing the amount of sleep you get will decrease the amount of food you crave. (No, it's not just because you can't eat while you're sleeping …) Research has shown that people who sleep less than 6 hours a night produce more of a hunger-inducing hormone and less of the hormone that balances your metabolism. You must be thinking this is the best weight loss system ever. You have just started and already I'm telling you to sleep more. See, I told you we'd get on just fine …

- **Am I dehydrated?** – Drink 8–12 glasses of water daily and drink a large glass of water 30 minutes before meals to satisfy your body and minimize your appetite. Often we are only thirsty when we think we feel hungry. Have a quick check in with yourself just now and count how many glasses of water or juice you had yesterday?

Quick check – How many glasses of water did you drink yesterday? ─────────────

Now, rate your emotional fatigue for yesterday on a scale from 1–10

1–2–3–4–5–6–7–8–9–10

Look again at how many glasses of liquid you had? Was it less than 8? If it was, then this is your most immediate task for today – Drink!

Tea and coffee don't count, neither do beer or wine. In the same way that chips don't count as one of your 5 portions of fruit and vegetables per day. Tea, coffee and alcohol dehydrate your body. Please drink lots of water, believe me this is one of the simplest and quickest ways to increase your energy levels, not to mention your concentration and general feeling of wellbeing. I'm sure your skin will thank you too. Drink, drink, drink. One of your journal entries for the next five weeks will be to log how many glasses of water you have had each day. How many have you had so far today?

- **Do I need more oxygen in my blood?** – Do you remember to breath? I know this might sound a little stupid but you'd be amazed the number of people who forget how important it is to breath properly. We can live without food for weeks, without water for days but only minutes without oxygen.

By learning to breathe properly, you can feed your body with this much needed nourishment. Breathing into the stomach, connecting to your diaphragm then breathing again … please take a few minutes to lie down or sit in a nice relaxing chair. Put one hand on your stomach (you'll need the other one to hold the book) and take a few nice deep breaths … Did your hand move? Did your stomach expand and contract in time with your breathing? If it did, well done! If not, then you are not breathing deeply enough. You may have noticed your chest expanding and contracting this is shallow breathing and is probably a result of you living in a state of stress.

I'm guessing that if this is the case you are feeling tight and tense. Try the exercise again until you can breath deeply into your stomach, really breath deeply; hold it for just a few seconds and then breath all the way out. Get as much oxygen as you can into your system and enjoy really breathing deeply for the next few minutes. You'll be amazed how relaxed and calm you will feel just by beginning to breath properly again.

- **Are you a fast eater?** Often when we overeat it's because we eat too quickly. Do you inhale your food? The body has an inbuilt mechanism to let you know when you've had enough, to let you know when you're full. The problem is that if we eat too quickly we don't notice we are full until it's too late. I had a friend at school who was very overweight. His Dad used to joke with him that he didn't eat till he was full he ate till he was tired. He simply didn't notice the signal telling him 'I'm full', He was too busy eating! So, in the same way you probably seldom feel hungry you probably seldom feel full.

I would imagine that you do feel stuffed though? A small design flaw in our make up is that it takes around 20 minutes for the signal to go from our body to our brain to let us know that we are full. If you are eating too quickly, you will not notice the signal to stop. If you don't get a signal to stop, how will you know? This is most commonly brought home to us at time of celebration like Christmas or Eid.

We all overeat. I think that's a given. Me included … but we rarely feel full when we are at the table, it's once we stop eating that it catches up on us and we slump down on the sofa absolutely stuffed! Does that sound familiar? It's not just at festival or celebration time either. If you eat too quickly, you'll miss the signal to stop! So, what I'd like you to do is to slow your eating speed all the way down … that's right, turn it all the way down (I'll reinforce this on the Slim Girl's Key Secret CD which you'll find in your Box of Secrets) but for now I just want you to make the conscious decision to eat much, much slower.

Eat slowly

Aim to halve the speed at which you normally eat. Put your knife and fork down between mouthfuls. This will slow you down and give you the chance to actually notice how full you are. The first thing you will notice is that you get full really quickly this way.

You'll also actually enjoy food much more as you'll be able to taste it properly, perhaps for the first time ever. However, there is a side effect of slowing down your eating. You will notice that some food tastes much better and some food tastes terrible! When you taste your food, (really taste your food) you will notice that fast food and ready meals actually don't taste very nice.

Don't take my word for it; try it the next time you eat. Slow down your eating speed and notice not only how your food really tastes but also how quickly you notice that you feel full … It never fails. Cutting down speed cuts down the amount you eat and here's the best bit … You will not be hungry! This is not about starving yourself, you'll eat till you're full then you stop. Perfect!

Next time you eat, take time to eat slowly; the funny thing is that it doesn't actually take much longer.. Well, you're not eating as much are you? So, take time to eat slowly and then just take another minute to jot down your findings in your journal. How much less did you eat compared with before? Enjoy feeling full and satisfied and then really enjoy that feeling of pride that you have left food on your plate … Really take pride in it, you owe it to yourself to break your old habits and feel good. If you take nothing else from this book, slowing down the speed at which you eat will make a dramatic difference.

Switch off 'emotional hunger'?

Am I really hungry or do I want to change the way I feel? I think I can safely say here that most overeating is emotional eating. We eat when we are happy, we eat when we are sad, we eat when we are sad and want to feel happy, we eat when we are stressed and want to feel calm, we eat when we are worried, we eat, we eat, we eat!

Now ... this is the cool part. It doesn't have to be this way. I have packed this book full of techniques, tips and tricks to break this habit and help you live a happy life with a balanced relationship with food. Quite possibly for the first time ever. Just take a moment for yourself. I know you're probably not used to doing that but just take a moment to think about if you are emotionally hungry?

If, at least one of the points above resonated with you then this is the book for you. I would guess that, for most people, at least 2 of the above would be true most days. Let me take you through a few quick tips to help you to eliminate emotional eating from your daily routine.

As I said earlier, most overeating is emotional eating. You are not alone. Overeating is not about logic it's about feelings, it's about emotions. If it were logical you would eat just as much as you need, then stop. End of story. After all you don't over fill your car with fuel or put too much washing powder in your machine. That would just be silly not to mention a waste ... So why is it that you reverse this when it comes to food? Too much petrol would spill out of the car and be a waste. So why is it that too much food which makes you spill out of your jeans is 'good, or thrifty or virtuous'? It just doesn't make sense at any logical level. Logically it doesn't work!

That's why diets alone don't work. You are not logical, you are a wonderful emotional human being but that in itself is part of the problem. We all eat emotionally and so I'm going to give you a few quick tips to make sure you can release yourself from emotional eating for good.

What if I told you that it only takes a few minutes to break the craving or habit for good? Easier said than done you may think … ! Well it's not.

If you've ever wondered how it is possible for people to change their mind in a heart beat then it's time to experience quick change for yourself. Change doesn't have to take a long time. Change happens very quickly, sure the procrastination usually takes a long time but change happens very quickly. Take a moment to just think of the number of times you have changed your mind and never gone back. Perhaps it was a relationship you decided was wrong for you or perhaps it was a job you resigned from because something happened which was the straw which broke the camel's back. Even that statement suggests that one thing can change the way we feel, that one last thing is enough to tip the balance and there's no going back.

So, why do we have to wait so long to make life changing choices? Well one reason is that we perceive them as BIG and big choices or changes can't be taken lightly and must involve some pain and suffering right? But ask yourself why? Why can't it just be easy to do what you know is right for you? There are a whole bunch of reasons why you might like to keep things as they are, even if you are unhappy. I have heard it many times that people just don't like change or are too old to change or that it's all very well for others but not for me. Whatever the reason, it is true that there is an inertia that has to be broken. Old habits and old ways of thinking can just lose their power as you read on and you can gain some new habits and keep them for good this time. The laws of inertia and momentum are simple. An object at rest wants to stay at rest whereas an object in motion wants to stay in motion. This is not my opinion, it's the Laws of Physics. The space shuttle uses most of its power getting off the ground but when it's orbiting at 17,500 miles per hour it hardly uses any power at all.

This is also true in the world of sport. As you know, I used to be a runner and it's a well known technique in speed endurance events to get out hard and fast. It's a lot of effort at the start but then you can shut down and cruise for as long as possible, saving energy and biding your time to kick for the finish.

So, back to you – Breaking the inertia can be easier than you think but you have to believe that it's possible and allow it to happen.

A few years ago I was filming a TV pilot for a "Face Your Fears" type of show where I was curing people of their animal phobias. During a break in filming I got chatting to the animal handler, a fascinating guy who, apart from not really liking animals (I suspect because his Dad was killed by the lion he was supposed to be 'taming'), was remarkable because he reckoned he could train any animal to do anything.

SLIM

Ok, I said, how do you can take a huge animal like an elephant and train it so that it won't run away when only a small rope and a chair restrains it? The answer, he said, was simple. 'The elephant doesn't know that it can escape. You see, the way they train elephants and many other large animals for that matter, is that from an early age they are tethered to an immovable object. Of course when they are young they try to pull against their shackles but, in time, they 'learn' that pulling is useless and they give up. They learn that when they are tethered there is no use in even trying to escape; they learn that they are helpless. They have 'learned to be helpless'.

One of the saddest stories I have heard to further illustrate this point is that of a bear in a zoo. The bear had been in his enclosure for many years and had spent most of his time walking round and round just inside the bars looking out at the outside world. As time went on and the regulation governing zoos changed, it was decided to enlarge the bear's pen. A new area was built, much larger than before, a far better environment for the old bear to live out his last years. When the new pen was finished the bear was sedated, the old bars were removed and the keepers retired to a safe distance and waited for the sleepy old bear to awaken to his new home. What happened next would bring a tear to a glass eye. The bear woke from his sleep, yawned and ... did nothing! For the whole of that day he remained in roughly the same place, a week later he still hadn't ventured further than a few meters from where he had slept. In fact, over the course of the next month the keepers observed that the bear remained within the area in which he had previously be caged, he even walked round in circles where the old bars had been. You see, the bear had lived in that environment for so long that he had 'learned' that the confines of its pen was the size of his world and that nothing existed outside that space so he didn't even try to venture further. There was nothing at all to hold him back. Nothing other than the idea the bear held in his mind of what was possible: the idea that he was trapped, that his life had always been that way so there was no use doing anything else.

Are you caged by your own limiting beliefs? Most of us to some extent, have an idea of what we are capable of. Of course, this idea of what we are capable of is just an idea in your mind based on your previous experience. You are caged by your own belief of what is possible.

What I need you to do now is to dare to dream, dare to wonder what might exist beyond the confines of your current thinking, beyond what you think you know. For this program to work for you, I need you to dream with me. You need to forget helplessness and become impatient and eager to see what you can do, what you can achieve. How far can you go now that nothing bars your way?

You'll remember when you were young you were probably into everything and keen to explore. As you got older you took a few knocks and 'learned' not to hope for too much, after all that way you'll not be disappointed. One of the biggest reasons why people don't start something is this 'fear of disappointment'. If you don't try, you'll not be disappointed but if you try and fail that'll hurt, right?

I need you to be brave for yourself again and dare to dream. Have faith in YOU and you'll not be disappointed, you'll be proud of yourself and be able to feel great in you, and about you again. Let's prove it to yourself that you deserve to be slim, fit and healthy. Are you up for it? I hope so, because I'm right here with you and so looking forward to receiving an email or picture from you when you've made some of your dreams come true. I'm hoping I'll be seeing a lot less of you very soon! Please keep in touch and let me know how you're getting on. You'll find me and many other people just like you on the forum pages at www.slimgirlsboxofsecrets.com

Ok – let's get going, I'm going to teach you a quick technique to let you break old habits and break that inertia to change. What do you crave? Craving is emotional hunger and many people find themselves giving in to their cravings and eating things that they don't really want, then feeling guilty about it afterwards. Sound familiar? Ok, well this might be a little strange but simple is often best. I'm about to introduce you to an amazing Thought Field Therapy Technique which will quickly eliminate cravings and give you control and choice again. You may have seen this technique demonstrated on TV by Paul McKenna, it's becoming quite well known as a quick way to re-set your emotional state. I learned this short cut version from Paul himself so just follow these simple steps ... the points you will be tapping on are

THE SLIM GIRL'S BOOK OF SECRETS

illustrated here but remember – I'll talk you through this on the accompanying CD.

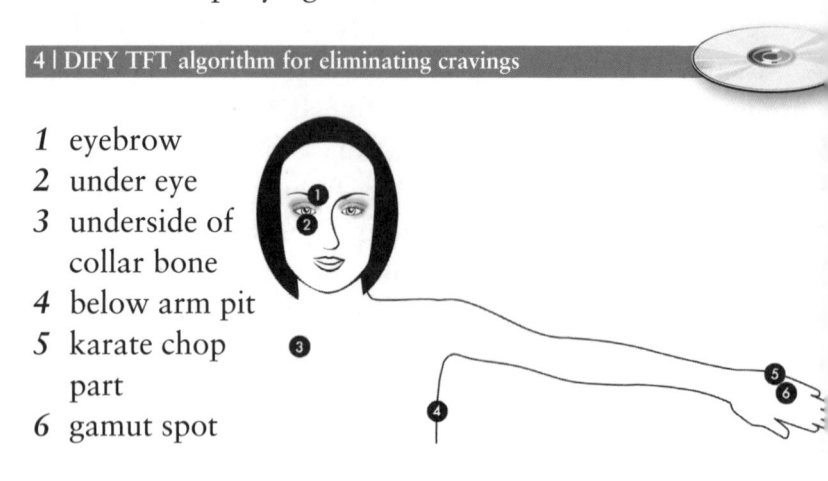

4 | DIFY TFT algorithm for eliminating cravings

1. eyebrow
2. under eye
3. underside of collar bone
4. below arm pit
5. karate chop part
6. gamut spot

Think about something that you normally can't resist. Tune in to the thought field (intentionally think about the craving you are removing).

Rate how upset you feel about the craving on a scale of 1–10 where 1= no craving at all and 10= the most compelled that you could possibly feel. Write down this rating here _____

1. Using 2 fingers of one hand, tap a spot at the beginning of the eyebrow, just above the bridge of the nose. Tap 5 times firmly.
2. Using 2 fingers of one hand, tap 5 times under the eye, about an inch below the bottom of the centre of the bony orbit high on the cheek. Tap firmly.

Tap the 'collar bone point' (to locate it take 2 fingers and run them down the throat to the top of the cen-

tre collarbone notch approximately where a man would knot his tie). From here move down one inch and then move to the right one inch. Tap this point 5 times.
4. Tap solidly 5 times under the arm about 4 inches below the armpit. On men this is level with the nipple and on women this is about the centre of the bra under the arm.
5. Find the PR spot. This is located on the outside edge of the hand between the wrist and the little finger. It is sometimes referred to as the karate chop part of the hand.
6. Tap mid way along this edge about 15 times using 2 fingers of the opposite hand.
7. Locate the gamut spot on the back of the hand, about 1 inch below the raised knuckles of the ring finger and the little finger when making a fist. Begin tapping the gamut spot with 2 fingers of the opposite hand, about 3 to 5 times per second while performing the 9 steps below.
8. Tap 5 or 6 times for each of the 9 exercises. It is very important to tap throughout all 9 exercises.
9. Close your eyes.
10. Open your eyes and look down to the left.
11. Look down to the right.
12. Whirl your eyes around in a circle in one direction.
13. Whirl your eyes around in a circle in the opposite direction.
14. Count ALOUD from 1–5 (it doesn't have to be loud but not into yourself).

THE SLIM GIRL'S BOOK OF SECRETS

15. Hum a few bars of a tune ALOUD.
16. Count aloud from 1–5 again.
17. Look at the floor.
18. Look at the ceiling.
19. Take another 1–10 rating.
20. To ensure that the improvements you've made are complete, hold your head level and move your eyes down then begin tapping the gamut point (back of your hand) as you move your eyes upwards.

I suggest that you take yourself off to the bathroom or somewhere quiet away from other people before you do this, otherwise you'll lose weight but it won't be much fun, it's hard to eat in a straight jacket ...! ☺ More information on TFT can be found at **www.tftrx.com**.

Practice this technique in the privacy of your own home before you try it out for real. Once you have it mastered it, it will take only a minute or so to do one complete sequence. What I have found is that when I work with clients using TFT, the craving or compulsion either halves in intensity each time you do it or it just drops completely. If you are one of the people for whom it halves just do it a couple of times till it's gone.

Make a note in your journal about how you get on with it and how many times you had to do it the first time to crack the craving. As with anything, practice makes perfect so keep at it. Physical action re-codes your neurology and then your brain can take over. In a good way now.

Slimming in Mind

The Power of Intention

I know you really want to make some big changes in your life but have you asked for it?

The mind is a funny thing. It has a mechanism for attracting what you focus on. It's almost as if you just have to ask and set the intention, then allow some space for what you've asked for to come into your life. It's all very well to say that you want it but you have to be flexible enough to allow the changes to happen. One of the biggest frustrations I have in my private client sessions is when people turn up and expect to be able to change their lives without actually changing anything in it. You need to be prepared to do things a little differently and that includes the way you allow yourself to think and be.

That's the key, it's the difference between dreaming or wishing and truly manifesting what you want. You may be familiar with *'The Secret'*, a movie and book by Rhonda Byrne? I would advise you, if you've not seen the movie or read the book to do so, just don't take it too seriously. In *The Secret*, some of the leading thinkers in the world of personal development point to the law of attraction as being 'the secret' which has been known and used for centuries by the great and the good to attract wealth and power into their lives. In my opinion, the secret falls slightly short of the real key to success. It is too shallow for my taste and I think it misses a key ingredient altogether.

SLIMMING IN MIND

The *real* secret is two fold: the law of attraction and the *choice* to take action. You see, simply wishing for a better life is obviously not the key. Don't you do that every day already? I'm sure you've already visualised yourself slim and healthy, driving that lovely car to a beautiful house where (insert hunk or babe of your choice) is running you a bath before declaring their undying love and leading you to the ... OK, OK that might just be in my head but you know what I mean ...

You open your eyes and find that nothing has changed and so you go to work and think 'it's not meant for me, nice idea but not meant for the likes of me'. Well, I've got news for you – the only person stopping you is you! I'm not being mean and blaming you here, you just haven't been shown another way yet.

Let me introduce you to a new way of being in the world. Weight loss is NOT logical, it's emotional. And, before you begin to lose pounds, you have to lose your old way of thinking and start to loosen your grip on the things that are holding you back. Once you are in a state of flow, you will find yourself being carried almost inexplicably towards your goals.

Now that leads me to the second part of the law of attraction: the choice of action. By action I do not mean the gym, or running, or aerobics or any other of the 'absolutely the best way to burn fat' exercises I'm sure you've tried already. I'm talking about the 'choice' of action. The first thing that I want you to do is to notice that you have 'choices'.

The cake may look nice but is it worth being fat for?

You have choice and choice gives you power. You have the choice about what you do or don't do. The choice about what you eat or don't eat. What you wear or don't wear and the choice about which actions you take. The important thing to do with choice is use it. Take action!

It's just a thought

You do not have the conscious choice over what you think! Let me say that again, just to be absolutely clear … You do not have the conscious choice over what you think. Thoughts happen independently of you. You obviously do think but you do not control it. Let me give you an example to make that distinction a little clearer … Think of your thoughts as being like television programmes, you do not have control over which programmes are shown but whichever one you choose to watch will be the one that will affect you. Just like with the television scenario you can choose which thoughts to engage with.

So just consider the possibility that;

Thoughts are just thoughts. It's the power 'you' give to them which dictates how they affect you and make you feel.

Just like with the TV, (where you can choose what you want to watch and which programmes just to skip past on your way to something better) so too you can choose which thoughts to engage with and which to just pass by. Let me stress this distinction. *Thoughts are just thoughts*. Research has shown that we each have around 50,000 of them every day. But it's actually more like the same 2,000 thoughts over and over again and just like with the TV you are not the programme controller. You are a bystander but you can choose which ones affect you and which you can just let go now.

This was brought home to me on a recent trip to New York. I was tired and jet lagged and couldn't sleep, so I put on the television. Four hundred channels and nothing on, not one show that caught my attention for the first 200-ish channels. I watched each for a second or two, made a quick judgement and then clicked on. Ruthlessly wielding my wand of power, flashing through the channels I eventually came across what looked like a financial life coaching show. (Yes, I am that much of a coaching geek). This is a show where people call in to speak to the host, tell her how much they earn, how much their outgoings are and what they would like to buy and she tells them whether they could afford it or not. I really got into it and found myself getting quite annoyed as I watched. I wasn't getting annoyed with the host or the callers but with the concept of the show, talk about giving your power to someone else! I'd like to say only on TV but actually we all do this every day of our lives. We allow things beyond our control (our thoughts) to dictate how we are in the world and how our world is for us.

After all '*it's just a thought*'. Thoughts pop into your mind every minute of every day, so much so that you do not even notice most of them. Then along come the ones *you* give power to and wham! You find yourself getting stuck into the pudding you didn't even want. When I ask my clients 'Why did you eat that …?' the most common answer is 'Once the thought came into my head I just had to have it' or 'As soon as I saw the menu something told me to have it'. Does this sound familiar? There are a million ways to say it but the general point is that if you have ever really wanted to eat something and felt totally compelled to do it then this section is for you. I suspect that means most people who read this book. This is definitely a section to turn the corner down on …

Thoughts create feelings and feelings create want.

We are absolutely chemically and socially conditioned to respond to our thinking. Once we get a thought in our mind we are conditioned to act on it. When we see something we want our brain releases a neuro transmitter chemical called Dopamine into our system which chemically causes us to 'crave' the object of our desire.

This is not just true for food, it is true of all consumables. Take a moment and play with your brain chemicals. Let's do a little science experiment on ourselves.

Just try playing with the thought of your favourite comfort food or some of the other things that you might also have a 'want' for. Just try on the idea of a chocolate or a special new pair of shoes, a new sports car, or a new designer handbag. Where did you get a feeling? Now let's make it even less specific and just use a brand name.

Try on the thought of Jimmy Choo or Chanel or Ferrari or Mulberry or Cadburys or Thorntons, bet you got a feeling then?

It's hardly a surprise, big name brands spend millions every year conditioning you to ensure that you get that feeling, then they associate their brand with your feelings. 'Feeling down?', A new pair of shoes will help, or 'Want to feel successful'? A new bag will do the trick or 'Need a hug?' 'How about some chocolate or a cake?' and so it goes on.

Then, when we actually get what we want we get another chemical released called 'Serotonin' the Happy Hormone. This goes on all the time. Once we have a desire, dopamine is there whether you like it or not and when you have that 'feel good' feeling you can bet that serotonin is calling.

Now I'm as much of a sucker for commercialism as anyone but when this addictive link between thoughts and actions is doing you harm, it's time to act.

(You can flip back to page 48 and tap away the feeling if you need to, for now it's ok).

It's just a thought but we're going to close down this little chemical tug of war, cut the rope and let you live the way 'you' want to for a change. I want you to imagine that we have a process which goes something like

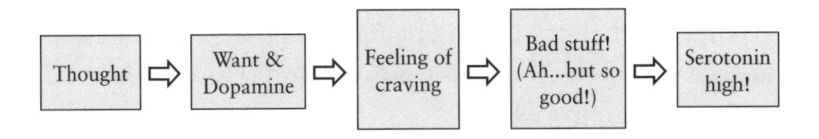

Thought ⇨ Want & Dopamine ⇨ Feeling of craving ⇨ Bad stuff! (Ah...but so good!) ⇨ Serotonin high!

The Serotonin high reinforces the idea that whatever it was that you had, did or ate made you feel good. So the next time you see it, you'll have the same thought. It's called anchoring and you'll learn how to collapse later.

(Now in your best 'Yoda' voice) "Thought leads to want, want leads to craving and craving leads to the dark side" ... Do you see how this works?

You are stuck in a vicious little chemical circle and it's all triggered by thought. Not for long ...!

The willpower method doesn't work or certainly not for very long and it's hard work because you are trying to break the link between 'craving' and 'action. It's too late by then but you know that already. Breaking the link between the feeling and the fridge alone doesn't work.

By the time you've got to this point you'll have thoughts, brain chemicals and cravings, not to mention years of conditioning all rushing you to a hot date with the fridge. This is where it all goes wrong ... I will help you to break this cycle much earlier (between thought and feeling) so you never get to the point where you feel like you're being driven by some universal force of craving.

It strikes me that almost every intervention I have come across whether it is for food, booze, cigarettes or any other kind of addictive behaviour tries to break the link between 'want' and 'action'. Why would you let it go that far then try to stop using will power? It's not Will power you need it's 'Won't power' and that comes much earlier in the process.

SLIMMING IN MIND

Let's be honest, if you don't have the desire for something you're not likely to do it, are you? Once you have the feeling of desire it's often too late. Sure there are things you can do that will take the craving away but you don't want to be constantly fighting against your feelings. I'm sure by now you're sick of that. So here's the secret …

Breaking this habit of reacting to thought is the first huge shift we're going to make. This alone may well be the key that changes your relationship with food and the way you are in the world forever …

I want you to get used to breaking this link and living on your terms for a change. How dare the program controller run your life? You may not be in control of your thoughts but you are in control of your actions … I hope you understand this distinction. If it's not clear yet, it will be as we move forward.

You have probably heard people say something like 'it's just a thought but …' You will hear me say that a lot from now on. 'It's just a thought'. We use that phrase all the time but I want you to get very familiar with it and to take it literally. When I say 'It's just a thought', that means it's just an idea or it's just an option or a channel you can choose to watch. Notice 'you' can choose. You can choose to engage or just flick on. Thoughts are just thoughts – you don't have to react to them. The technique and principles I am about to teach you have been used to treat drug addiction, abusive behaviour, stress, depression and I can honestly say have been one of the biggest breakthroughs in my own life. Conventional therapy focuses on change from the outside, looking at how something outside you can change you and your behaviour. If you think about psychology, all talking therapies and even medicine, you'll find that in all of these fields the agent of change is on the outside. Whether it's the therapist, the techniques (as with TFT) or the medication, the agent of change is on the outside. I hope that makes sense? The radical breakthrough I had was realising that change is an inside out process. You change on the inside first, then live that change on the outside.

5 | DIFY – Just sitting

The exercise around this could not be simpler ... It can be found in Peter Fenner's book *Radiant Mind* if you want to read further about it.

I want you to find somewhere comfortable, sit down and close your eyes and just sit. Sounds too easy doesn't it? You probably think I've lost my marbles. I'm supposed to be helping you to lose weight and get fit and yet I've just asked you to sit down and put your feet up. On the other hand you might be thinking 'This is the best weight loss program ever'! Let me explain ... In exactly the same way as you can choose to watch a TV channel or not, you can choose to focus on or react to a thought if 'you' want to. You don't have to and here we are going to break the link between thoughts and actions.

I'd love it if you just took a moment or two now to put the book down, close your eyes and 'Just Sit'. Do nothing except let a thought come to mind, then *let it go*. Another one will replace it and I want you to just let that go too … Keep going, just let thoughts come to mind and then let them to go. Sounds easy and it is if you allow it to be but it's very effective. You don't put the thoughts there, just allow whatever thoughts show up to come to mind and then just allow them to go … do that for a few minutes now, then come back to the book and we'll be ready to move on …

Ok, I hope you didn't fall asleep. Let me just check a few things … How did your thoughts show up for you? Do you think in pictures? Are your thoughts like a little voice in your head? Do you see the words you are thinking? However, they show up for you, just notice how this worked for *you*. As we go forward you will notice that there appears to be a gap or distance opening up between you and your thinking, almost as if you are becoming separated from your thoughts and you can just notice them go by.

Whichever way your thoughts are represented to you, you will probably notice this type of separation. It might take a bit of practice (for me it took about a week of 'just sitting' for 20 minutes every day to get the benefit and to start noticing that I wasn't simply reacting to my thoughts anymore). That said, I have just done this with a friend and in just a few minutes she was feeling happier and a lot less cluttered.

That's all very well you might think, but what's it got to do with my waistline? Well, I'll share with you a very real food example that happened to me just last weekend. I was out for lunch with some friends and had just enjoyed a wonderful meal in a fabulous restaurant on the banks of Loch Lomond. I've often thought it would be easier to lose weight if we lived in a warm climate (after all, who wants to eat salad when it's cold, wet and rainy?)

Obviously, this is just a story we tell ourselves as a reason why we want the warm, sweet comfort food. It may feel very real but it's just another thought. You only have to look at the obesity statistics for California (where the weather is considerably better for salad munching) to realise that it's just a story we tell ourselves. Anyway, the weather on Sunday was about as far away from salad munching as it's possible to get, so when the subject of dessert was raised it seemed 'obvious' that we would all have one. I'm not really a habitual pudding eater but I do have a sweet tooth and can scoff my comfort food with the best of them. So – who's for dessert? I scanned down the menu where I found apple crumble calling out to me. I got that familiar feeling in my chest and, for a moment, I really wanted it … then it passed. I didn't do anything but something happened and the thought just didn't have any power anymore. I thought about it and decided NOT to have pudding (much to everyone's astonishment I have to say). Then something else happened, the others started at first to make suggestions of puddings I would like (more to appease their own guilty feelings than out of any genuine concern for my wellbeing I suspect). But no, the thought had gone and it was no good. I didn't want pudding. Can you guess what happened next?

That little gap (caused by me pausing and then saying no) gave my friends enough time to 'choose' that they didn't actually want a dessert either ... not one of them ordered pudding!

All this happened in a matter of a minute or so but not one of us had dessert. Now, I don't expect you to keep your friends waiting until they decide they don't want to eat anything, but the cool observation for me is that just having a break between thought and action gives freedom of choice.

I left the restaurant with no feeling of loss, no thoughts of 'I wish I had ...', in fact no thoughts of food whatsoever. I had not argued or talked myself out of it. I had not thought of all the positive benefits of not eating dessert. I had simply allowed myself (unconsciously I must add) time to choose instead of reacting.

This approach can be applied to so many areas of your life but for now we'll stick to weight loss.

Just Sitting again ...
Your mission, should you choose to accept it, is to do nothing for 20 minutes every day. I know that you probably immediately came up with a whole bunch of thoughts why you can't – kids, work, husband, no time. 'He must be joking, has he seen my life?' No – but I've seen thousands just like it. Even if it's just the 20 mins before you turn out the light at the end of the day, I want you to find time, sit down, close your eyes and do noth-

ing. Do not deliberately think of anything. Just allow thoughts to come into your mind (remember you don't control these anyway). When they come to mind, just let them go. 'It's just a thought' – so let it go. It might feel a little strange at first, but it is new to you so, of course, it's going to feel a little odd. It'll take a little time, but soon it'll feel like second nature to you. As you do it day by day, you will notice changes. It might initially be in the way you experience your own thoughts, then the connection or lack of connection between you and your thinking and then you will begin to notice the disconnection between your thoughts and your actions. This is the cool part – you can choose what to watch, what to let go and what to take part in. On your terms.

It's about living your life on your terms.

6 | DIFY Getting used to just sitting.

Please 'just sit' for 20 minutes every day for the next week. That's all. Only 20 minutes to a new way of thinking and being in the world. Are you up for it? Great, then set a timer for 20 minutes. You'll probably have one on your mobile phone or, if like my Mum you can't work it, just set the oven timer and go with that.

Close your eyes. Don't deliberately think of anything, just quieten your mind and *allow* thoughts to come to mind, then let them go. Remember thoughts turn up differently for everyone, some as pictures, others hear words like a little voice within and others see the actual words themselves. Play around with how best to let thoughts go. Maybe, for you, it's just to let them pass through or maybe they dissolve away or fade into the distance. Find whichever way works for you and do that. There is no right or wrong way, only what works for you.

Ok let's do a quick recap –

Set your mind on success – Listen to The Slim Girl's Key Secret CD accompanying this book to effortlessly program your mind for success. The only thing you have to do to ensure your success is make a little time to focus on yourself and make some small changes. Allow yourself to be flexible and attract good things into your life.

Just sit for 20 minutes each day – This is most people's favourite part. Just sit and notice your thoughts until you find that you are not habitually reacting to thought and instead have the choice to pick and choose your actions.

Drink plenty of water – 8 glasses per day will have you feeling more energised and healthier. Don't forget that your skin will love you for it too.

Eat slowly – Slow your eating speed all the way down so that you actually taste your food and notice when you are feeling full. It'll be quicker than you are used to and you might surprise yourself with just how little food you need.

Remember to breath – Tension and stress can cause your breathing to become too shallow. Take a few really nice deep breaths in, hold for a few seconds and breath all the way out. Get into the habit of doing this any time you feel tense.

Emotionally hungry – tap it away! Remove cravings if you have them by tapping them away. We are all emotional human beings, why should you be any different? You can have emotions without linking them to food though. Any time you have a craving or an emotional urge (for anything) that you do not want you can simply tap it away.

Only eat when you are physically hungry – Check in with your stomach and ask if you are physically hungry, not ravenous, but nicely hungry is the best time to eat – slowly remember.

Leaving food = feeling good – How good will it feel to know you have broken the old 'clear your plate programming' by leaving food and feeling good about it. You have the chance to find out every mealtime.

Sleep! (my favourite ☺) – A good sleep at night will benefit you far more than you know. Aim for 8 hours each night and enjoy feeling refreshed. This is your time to recover and refresh. Enjoy it.

SLIMMING IN MIND

In the next section we are going to explore how you can get a bit fitter, have more energy, burn fat quicker and generally have a bit of fun in the process …

Fit

Before you go any further in this section, if you are in any doubt about whether you are able to participate in any exercise programs please consult your doctor first. It's not strenuous but better safe than sorry.

In this section you will learn all about the massive benefits exercise can have on your life, not only to your shape but also on your metabolism, energy levels, your whole outlook on life and many others which I will tell you about later. By simply making a little exercise part of your life, you will feel amazing, enjoy the physical results, reap the many benefits to your body both internally and emotionally and never look back. I promise.

As you know already I do know a little bit about this subject. That said, the world of fitness has moved on such a long way in recent years. For the most part it has become more efficient, exercises have been developed that give you a much greater return for your effort. Now I'm all for that and I'm sure you want to get the most benefit for any effort you put in, so I have teamed up with one of the very best personal trainers I have ever met. I actually trained her years ago but she has gone on to enhance her skills, developed her own style and now she's the one putting me through my paces … How did that happen? Anyway, she's brilliant and you'll be in very good hands. Alba and I have developed this plan to be bang up to date with all the moves that will help you to tone up and strip away body fat faster than you can believe. Don't worry we'll guide you through it and take it very gently.

The real question we need to ask ourselves is "Can I afford not to exercise?" Most of us don't exercise at all, never mind enough and experts say that our levels of inactivity have become so bad, we are seriously threatening our health. With a little help from this program and all the simple and effective advice in it, you can do something about that and it's never too late to start!

This is the first day of the rest of your life moving towards a slim, **fit**, healthy and active YOU!!.

Exercising and becoming fit doesn't mean you need to train to run a marathon or look like a body builder, it's about what you want to achieve and, more importantly, about having fun – you don't have to be a hardcore gym junkie. In fact I'd really prefer it if you weren't.

Before I go on to suggest types of exercises and why I have chosen them, let's start at the beginning. Let me tell you about the many positive effects exercise can have on your life – these alone should have you dashing for your trainers and t-shirt! Think of exercise as grown up playtime!! (No kiss chase allowed though – at least not in your first week, you'll need to build up your fitness so you can catch your target!! ☺)

Benefits of Exercise on your Energy Levels

I think this is a perfect place to start, as many of my clients come to me and say they are too tired to exercise in the first place. Even though their jobs don't require them to be physically active, they still feel very tired at the end of the day and don't have the energy to exercise.

THE SLIM GIRL'S BOOK OF SECRETS

So here's the cool bit, when you start to exercise, your body starts to naturally release chemicals which give you that good feeling and uplifting emotions. These are called endorphins (think of these as 'them dolphins').

When you exercise 'them dolphins' start swimming around your body, splashing you on the inside with sparkles of energy and good feelings. This happens naturally but we can help them dolphins by dipping in and connecting to them now.

7 | DIFY – Them sparkly dolphins.

I'd like you to take a few moments to close your eyes and make still your mind. If you've ever swam in the Caribbean at night, you may be familiar with the type of algae that reflects the moonlight? It looks like stars in the night sky, only it's in the water. If you've not had the pleasure, just imagine a clear night sky filled with stars and then flip the picture upside down. Now, I'd like you to close your eyes and take a dip and swim in the stars and sparkles and let them dance around you like little flecks of sparkly magic, each one is a sparkle of a dream and a little part of you. Invite them in and let them fill your body. Then just go inside and explore your body from the inside (not literally), just imagine going down inside your body and taking a tour around, spreading sparkles of good feelings like glittering confetti glistening in the moonlight. That sparkle is always within you, all you have to do is to allow it to flourish and enjoy the great feeling that can spread through your body, just like 'them dolphins' splashing and dancing. You can't help but let go and feel good!

This exercise in itself gives you more energy and when we feel good we naturally feel more energetic. Anytime you're feeling sluggish, just call those dolphins for help.

By exercising, you are also increasing the amount of blood and oxygen carried to your heart, muscles and other vital organs. This speeds up your metabolism and burns more fat than usual (which we will cover in more depth later on), this in turn also increases your energy levels. By having increased muscle strength and energy, your body will be working at peak efficiency causing your energy levels to really soar – WOW! Doesn't that sound much better!! Everyday things will become easier to do and we could all do with a bit of that ... Sorry, if I'm sounding too cheesy here, I'm just doing my motivational bit ... Tee Hee!

Benefits on Metabolism

Fancy losing weight while sitting on the couch? Too right!

I think this is the one factor that most people want to hear about – we want to know how exercising is going to help us to lose weight and work its magic even when we are sitting at our desks or watching television. When you know that magic is happening inside even while you rest, you'll find this is always a great motivation to push yourself just a little bit harder.

A simple explanation of Metabolism is the amount of energy (calories) your body burns to maintain just itself. Your body is constantly burning calories, whether you are eating, sleeping, working or exercising. When you exercise you will burn more calories than when you are sleeping, but your body is a furnace which is constantly burning energy, 24 hours a day, it never stops.

Our metabolic rate is affected by our body composition and, by this, I mean the amount of muscle you have in comparison to the amount of fat. Muscle uses calories to maintain itself. If you are more muscular (and have a lower fat percentage) you are said to have a higher metabolism than others that are less muscular. For example, let's say there are two women.

Annie
10 Stone (64kg)
Doesn't exercise
High percentage of body fat (35% or 22kg)
Low level of lean muscle (65% or 42kg)
Annie has a lower metabolism.

Beth
10 Stone (64kg)
Exercises on a regular basis
Low level of body fat (20% or 13kg)
High level of lean muscle (80% or 51kg)
Beth has a higher metabolism.

Beth does a combination of weight bearing exercises and aerobic activities (walking, jogging, swimming, etc). During aerobic exercise, the focus is on burning calories and working her cardiovascular system (heart and lungs). This speeds up her metabolism during the activity and even when she has stopped.

When she is doing her weight bearing exercises, or other resistance work, she is creating more lean muscle. Lean muscle burns more calories not only during the exercise but continuously, even when she is doing other things.

To explain further, for every 1 kg of extra lean muscle that Beth has, she is burning approximately an extra 25 calories a day doing absolutely nothing. Comparing her to Annie shows that, even though they are exactly the same weight, Beth burns an extra 225 calories every single day, as she has 9 kg more lean muscle than Annie. This sends her metabolism through the roof and makes her body a fat burning furnace, burning more calories even when she is sitting on the couch.

So, in summary, one of the top ways to keep your metabolism fired up is to EXERCISE!!

Muscle, unlike fat, is metabolically active – it burns calories. So, by increasing your lean muscle, even when you are "just sitting" you will be burning more calories and losing weight!

Benefits on your Body Shape and Body Confidence

So now you know the science behind the exercise but will that keep you motivated? Most of us don't really care about the reasons exercise improves our metabolic rate. What we want to see, and what will keep us even more motivated, is the changes it will have externally on our shapes and our confidence.

Let's face it, we all want to look and feel good about our bodies and ooze confidence. This is not about striving to be super skinny, it's to be able to look in the mirror and think "Wow, I do look good!" It's about getting yourself to a realistically healthy level that is right for you and not about putting yourself under any pressure to get there. Just enjoy the journey and, before you know it, you will be hearing the compliments and feeling great!

Or, if you're already there, brilliant!! It's just about getting a better quality of life by incorporating some exercise into it.

Ok, I'm hoping that I have convinced you exercise is a great way to supercharge your body and a great tool for weight loss.

Now the number one question is "What types should I do and how will they help me to change my body shape and give me confidence?" Ok that's really 3 questions, but who's counting?

This is where Alba and I have really focused on and have designed the programme that's going to work best for you.

When you are doing aerobic / cardiovascular exercise you are burning calories. The more of this type of exercise you do, the fitter you will become, which will enable you to exercise more effectively and burn even more calories as you go. Also, the fitter you are, the more efficient your muscles will become at using fat for energy. This is why someone who is fit finds it relatively easy to stay lean.

Weight bearing resistance exercise also burns calories while increasing muscle mass, strength, endurance and tone. I'm not talking about sweating buckets in the gym, but just run with me on this.

A lot of women are reluctant to introduce weight bearing exercises into their normal routine as they think they will get big muscles and resemble a body builder. Let me reassure you, this is not the case. Muscle building in women is really difficult to achieve, even with a specifically tailored programme, but what you can get with resistance work is a lean, sculpted body to die for that not only looks hot but burns energy quickly and efficiently, making it easy to maintain.

The way resistance exercise works is that initially it puts the muscle under stress, which causes the muscle to have to repair itself and in doing so become stronger and leaner. "I think that the fact that all this is going on in your body and at the same time you are burning calories and fat and changing shape is truly amazing – personally, it has me reaching for my trainers and wanting more!" Alba said that, not me …☺ But a little bit done consistently and well goes a very long way.

With aerobic exercise the main focus is on burning calories whilst working your heart and lungs. As you burn more calories and fat you will lose body fat resulting in your body starting to change shape and tone. Aerobic exercise also releases adrenaline and serotonin, remember, I mentioned this one earlier? It's that same chemical that makes you happy and with all of that going on you can guarantee that your confidence will go through the roof.

Gaining control of your body size and weight through fitness is also an amazing way to increase self-esteem. You look better and are more confident, which empowers you in everything you do. You will find that the motivation and psychological changes made through regular exercise spills over into other areas of your life and you will be better able to make other necessary and desirable changes. Imagine trying on that size 12 dress and it actually fitting (and not having to hold your breath and suck in your tummy to make it 'fit') ☺.

Health Benefits

Some of the other benefits you really need to know about are the health related ones. Whilst a lot goes on to increase our metabolism, lose weight and fat, to change our body shape and increase confidence, one of the most important set of benefits are those to our general health. Of course, this is a slimming book but it is a lot wider than that. I genuinely want you to be slim, fit, healthy and active. Exercise has given me so much in my life, both physically and emotionally, I'd love you to feel the same. I'm not talking about heading off to the gym to pose in the latest gear, though you're very welcome to, if that's what takes your fancy. I'm not a member of a gym and frankly have no desire to join one. I exercise at home or go for a walk or run outside in the fresh air. Similarly, this program does not require you to go to the gym or even leave the house to enjoy some of the health benefits of a little bit of exercise.

Reduces blood pressure

While you exercise, your arteries and capillaries dilate, which boosts circulation. If you exercise regularly, you can benefit from reduced blood pressure, lower your risk of a heart attack and improve any circulatory problems.

Reduces stress

The worries and stresses of everyday living (commuting, work demands, family conflicts, money worries, etc.) are common to us all. Exercising can set you up for the day and make sure you are ready to tackle anything that comes your way. It will help to keep you focused and increase your concentration levels. Exercise straight after work is the perfect natural therapy that can release you from the stress of work and change your mood for the better.

You will sleep better too! Exercise in the middle of the day and you'll relieve any of the morning stress and leave you set up for the afternoon (increased blood flow to the brain will allow you to think more clearly which will help with problem-solving). If you are fitter, you will be able to handle pressure and stress from your daily job or life better than when you were unfit.

Exercise is one of the best ways to relieve stress and can be described as nature's Prozac. The release of those little chemicals, endorphins and serotonin, are the body's feel-good hormones, and nothing improves your mood and suppresses depression better than a bit of exercise. Just 20 minutes will make all the difference.

Relieves PMS symptoms

For women, exercising can help relieve the pain, improve your mood and reduce stress and tension. Some experts believe that women with more PMS problems have lower endorphin levels, so this makes exercise a particularly effective treatment to relieve the symptoms and restore a natural balance. Have you noticed a theme of 20 mins yet? No time at all but it will make a huge difference.

Benefit in combating osteoporosis

Osteoporosis is a thinning of the bones that occurs over time for most people but is most common in women over the age of 50. Evidence shows that weight-bearing exercise helps build and maintain bone density. Studies have shown bone density increases by doing regular resistance exercises 2 or 3 times a week. This type of weight bearing exercise stimulates bone formation and retains calcium in the bones that are bearing the load, making them denser and stronger. A University of Arkansas study shows that 2 percent of college-age women already have osteoporosis. A further 15 percent have sustained significant losses in bone density and may be well on their way to developing the disease, so it's something you should definitely take action on. Any exercise that places a force on a bone will strengthen it, thereby helping to reduce the effects of osteoporosis.

The benefits I have mentioned above are probably the most important and topical but there are still a whole lot more, some of which I have listed below. I did a quick search in the web to pull together this list. Be impressed, be very impressed. Some of these I didn't even know were possible …

- Improves digestion
- Reduces your risk of diabetes
- May help to reduce the risk of cancer
- Enhances quality of sleep
- Adds a sparkle and radiance to complexion
- Improves body shape
- Tones and firms muscles
- Helps you gain strength without bulk
- Provides more muscular definition
- Enables weight loss and keeps it off
- Makes you more supple
- Burns extra calories
- Improves circulation and helps reduce blood pressure
- Increases lean muscle tissue in the body
- Improves appetite for healthy foods

- Alleviates menstrual cramps
- Alters and improves muscle chemistry
- Increases metabolic rate
- Enhances coordination and balance
- Improves posture
- Eases and possibly eliminates back problems and pain
- Makes the body use calories more efficiently
- Lowers resting heart rate
- Increases muscle size through an increase in muscle fibres
- Improves body composition
- Increases body density
- Helps to decrease fat tissue more easily
- Makes body more agile
- Is the greatest body tune-up
- Reduces joint discomfort
- Enriches sexuality (takes practice … after all, you've got to be match fit)
- May add a few years to life (you may get your telegram from the Queen – although there may not be many bedroom antics by this point match fit or not!!)
- Increases your range of motion
- Enhances immune system
- Improves glycogen storage
- Enables the body to utilize energy more efficiently
- Increases enzymes in the body which burn fat
- Increases concentration of myoglobin (carries oxygen in muscles) in skeletal muscles
- Enhances oxygen transport throughout the body

- Improves liver functioning
- Increases speed of muscle contraction and reaction time
- Enhances feedback through the nervous system
- Strengthens the heart
- Improves blood flow
- Helps to alleviate varicose veins
- Increases maximum cardiac output
- Increases contractility of the heart's ventricles
- Increases the weight and size of the heart
- Improves contractile function of the whole heart
- Makes calcium transport in the heart and body more efficient

Are you impressed yet?

There's 50 reasons to get you moving and start living!!
☺ Remember

"It's not about the amount of days in your life but the amount of life in your days"

Having really highlighted and explained all the benefits that exercise can bring into your life I'm sure you're now ready to get started. So, get your trainers on and let's get going.

On your marks …

In this section we'll talk a little about types of exercise and explain the exercises we have chosen for you, then introduce you to a 5 week training plan which will give you that kick start and fire up your fitness and motivation levels.

THE SLIM GIRL'S BOOK OF SECRETS

Our aim is to make exercise a permanent part of your life and, for this purpose, I want you to think about your exercise sessions as playtime, your time to have fun, lose your inhibitions, shake your booty, strut your stuff and let getting in shape be the natural side effect.

The key to effectively incorporating exercise into your life is that familiar phrase 'little and often'. There's no need to sweat it out at the gym for 2–3 hours every day. If you do 20–30 minutes of exercise 3–5 times a week and ensure that you are following a healthy nutritional plan, this will be enough for you to start to feel and see a significant change both internally and externally.

How will you know you're doing well?

Monitoring the changes and your progress is important, but don't forget to look for the more subtle markers of success. Remember we're not going to get hung up on scales and weight, this can be detrimental to self-esteem and confidence. Go by the feelings of wellbeing you get from exercising, by noticing that you'll start to have more energy and body confidence. The knock on effects from this will be noticing your clothes getting a little looser and seeing how your body changes shape and tones up.

I've had so many clients who were really happy with how they were starting to look and feel and then they jump on the scales and maybe have put on a pound or two and it's as if all their other achievements are worthless.

I personally think that scales should come with a mental health warning. But everyone is different and, if you are more motivated by scales and actually seeing the changes in number form, then go for it but just weigh yourself on a weekly basis or wait longer if you can (definitely not every day) as your weight can fluctuate from one day to the next for many reasons and sometimes you may find you weigh more even though you are doing everything right.

One possible reason for this is that muscle is heavier than fat. Therefore your weight may stay the same or increase a little but if you can feel that your clothes are getting loose, this means that you are losing body *fat* which is more important than just weight loss. If you think about it, you want to be slim not light, it's your size and shape that matters.

Types of Exercise

The following training plan is suitable for everyone and should be progressed week by week as you become fitter and feel the need to challenge your body a bit more. There is a mix of strength/resistance exercise to help tone and shape your body and short burst cardiovascular moves to get your heart and lungs really working and burn more fat for a good all round workout that is so simple to follow but really effective. And you can do it from the comfort of your own home.

The main exercises we have chosen are using the body's major muscle groups (chest, legs and back). Blasting these will help to achieve firm, toned curves in all the right places! This will also ensure you get a good workout and make you look leaner and stronger. It's all too tempting for all of us to focus only on those 'trouble spots' like your stomach, thighs or bum. Don't just take my word for it though let's get some medical input, 'You'll see lots of exercise programs, devices and machines in television commercials that claim to get rid of fat from your belly. While they can strengthen your belly muscles, there is no such thing as spot reduction. Well, not without surgery, and we're not going there.

When you take in more calories than your body burns, you store them as fat. Some people store fat primarily in their hips and are thought to be at a lower risk for heart attacks and diabetes, while others who store their fat primarily in their bellies are at an increased risk for heart attacks and diabetes. You store more that half the fat in your body underneath your skin and over your muscles. Exercising a muscle does not get rid of fat over the specific muscles that are exercised. If it did, tennis players would have less fat in their racquet arms, but they don't.

Exercises and "ab" machines can strengthen sagging belly muscles but they will not remove extra fat from your belly. The only way to lose fat from the place where you store most of your fat (whether it's your belly or your hips) is to lose weight overall'.

Let me call in an expert here.

Dr Gabe Mirkin – A practicing physician for more than 40 years and a radio talk show host for 25, Dr. Mirkin is a graduate of Harvard University and

Baylor University College of Medicine. He has written 16 books and completed over 40 marathons so he knows a thing or two about it.

The best means of achieving a lean, strong and proportioned body is to work your upper and lower body evenly. By using all the major muscle groups, your heart will be working more effectively as it will need to pump a larger volume of blood to these areas. This will result in you burning more calories and fat! If you just worked an individual muscle such as your inner thigh or biceps, you would need to do a lot more exercises to burn the same amount of calories as working the whole of your legs or chest. So by doing it my way you get a bigger return for the effort put in!! Now that sounds like a good deal to me! If you're going to do it, you might as well do it the smart way!

Get set ...

Motivation and momentum

Remember the key secret with exercising is to do little and often, keep up your enthusiasm and motivation and you **will** see results. If you keep seeing results you'll keep up your momentum. It really is a case of keep doing little and often and you will notice a big difference. Most people give up just before they start to see a benefit. This is not a quick fix scheme. This is about making small changes that you can make part of your daily routine as easily as brushing your teeth or doing your hair. It's a funny thing but I'll bet you wouldn't dream of leaving the house with wild hair and your clothes needing ironing. So why not take the same meticulous care with your size, shape and health? I have found that there really is a funny rule about time management. If you want the time, you'll find the time. It's a bit like when you get a really good book and somehow you find the time to read it, despite the fact that you are just as busy as you have always been. Actually I'm learning that it's the same with writing a book. If you want the time, you'll find the time and it's time for you to start living your values and taking better care of yourself!!!

Be Realistic

Concentrate on easy, effortless daily exercise and food habits and the rest will follow. It's not a race, have fun and enjoy the journey. This is about making incremental changes that will help you move gradually towards better health and a better body. Establish good habits but, of course the **occasional** indulgence is fine and even encouraged. You have to live and this is not one of those "go live in a monastery" books – it's about getting more out of your life.

Measure your success and jot it down in your journal. Note down when your clothes are feeling looser or when you put on an outfit you haven't been able to fit into for a while. Make your goal to get back into that dress you bought last summer or those favourite jeans.

Hurry up and take your time

Take your time with the routines and exercise to begin with. Learn the correct techniques before you start. Build up as you start to feel more confident with the exercises and, as you feel fitter, you can increase duration and intensity. Remember this is **your** workout so take it at your own pace.

To monitor how hard you're working on all of your workouts, use an RPE scale (rate of perceived exertion). This is based on a scale of 1 to 10 with

- *1* being calm and relaxed when you started,
- *4* is "comfortable but you can feel you're working",
- *7* "you can talk but must stop talking (or singing to the music) to catch your breath"
- *10* means "the hardest thing you've ever done".

A good idea to begin with is to stay between 6 or 7 out of 10 and, as you get fitter and feel more comfortable, you push yourself a little more.

GO !

The cunning plan

Below I have outlined the plan as a whole and then explained the techniques of the exercises, the number of times each exercise should be performed, the number of times the routine should be completed (depending on how much time you have), how the warm up and cool downs help and finally how you can progress and add

THE SLIM GIRL'S BOOK OF SECRETS

Week	Day 1	Day 2	Day 3	Day 4	Day 5	Day 6	Day 7
1	Sculpt and blast workout	Rest	Any CV exercise. Powerwalk, jog, swim or cycle 15–20 mins	Rest	Sculpt and blast workout	Rest	Active rest, i.e. walking dogs/washing car/brisk walk/gardening
2	Sculpt and blast workout	Rest	Any CV exercise. Powerwalk, jog, swim or cycle. 20–25 mins	Rest	Sculpt and blast workout	Rest	Active rest, i.e. walking dogs/washing car/brisk walk/gardening
3	Sculpt and blast workout	Rest	Any CV exercise. Powerwalk, jog, swim or cycle. 25–30 mins	Rest	Sculpt and blast workout	Rest	Any CV exercise. Powerwalk, jog, swim or cycle. 25–30 mins
4	Sculpt and blast workout	Rest	Sculpt and blast workout	Any CV exercise. Powerwalk, jog, swim or cycle. 30–35 mins	Sculpt and blast workout	Rest	Any CV exercise. Powerwalk, jog, swim or cycle. 30–35 mins
5	Sculpt and blast workout	Rest	Sculpt and blast workout	Any CV exercise. 35–40 mins	Sculpt and blast workout	Rest	Any CV exercise. 35–40 mins

more exercises from the pick and mix section if you feel ready.

You'll find all the exercise moves and routines on your workout DVD 2. It might be an idea to pop it on now and take a look. Each exercise is explained and then joined up in the routine for you to follow along with at home.

All that you'll need
A little space: You don't want to be breaking that valuable china or crashing into your furniture. Make sure you have room to move.
Suitable kit: Bring on the lycra and leg warmers – or something to keep you cool and don't forget those trainers (the ones you made a mad dash for earlier and are holding in your hand since I started talking about metabolism and losing body fat, ok maybe not?). But you don't want to be slipping especially on wooden floors, so go and get them now, they'll also give you cushioning when doing the aerobic/cardio moves.
Music: Something that'll get you motivated and has a good strong beat.
Equipment: A chair or sofa, some water bottles or cans of soup/beans.
Water: Keep hydrated. By now you should be well used to enjoying the benefits of drinking (water) regularly. If you're using water bottles as weight then no drinking from those! Get yourself another one, I'm wise to you, no cheating!

Fresh air: If possible, try and exercise near an open window.

The workout

I'm firstly going to run through the sections in the workout and what each one means for you.

Warm up:

Warming up your body, increasing your heart rate and getting your joints moving so your body and muscles are ready to exercise. The warm up is essential, not warming up the body is a bit like someone dumping you into a cold shower in the morning without warning – that's what you would be doing to your muscles and body if you just went straight into the routine. OUCH!!

The Routine:

The main workout will consist of a mixture of strengthening and toning moves using your major muscles groups combined with short burst cardio moves to raise the intensity and get your heart and lungs fired up.

Cool-down and stretch:

Easing the intensity and stretching for muscle lengthening and toning.

Are you ready to begin? Pop on the DVD now ...

Lycra on??	CHECK or any clothing that will keep you cool ☺
Trainers on?	CHECK
Music on??	CHECK
Bean cans ready ??	CHECK

LETS GO!!
Remember to keep your tummy muscles pulled in tight throughout the workouts so you're giving your abdominals a good workout too!!

Sculpt and blast routine !!
Warm up
Perform each one for approx 1 min. You should feel warm and slightly out of breathe by the end of your warm up.

Step 1
Marching on the spot – for 1 min

Step 2
Side step – stepping from side to side

Step 3
Increasing intensity
Wide side steps and adding arms back and forth – as feet come together at the side, drive arms back and forth.

THE SLIM GIRL'S BOOK OF SECRETS

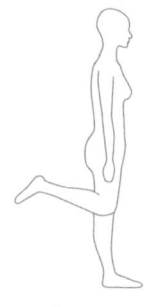

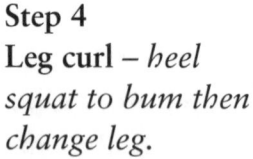

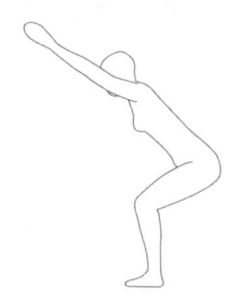

Step 4
Leg curl – *heel squat to bum then change leg.*

Step 5
Squats with arms overhead – *as you sit back drive your arms over your head.*

Step 6
Standing Hamstring stretch – *take one leg in front of you, bend the other leg and push your bottom back with hands on the bent knee, push your tail bone backwards and you will feel a stretch in the back of the thigh of the straight leg.*

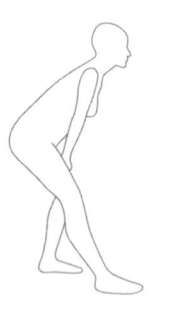

Step 7

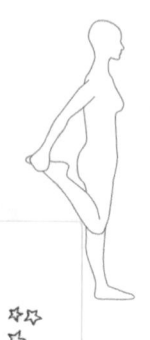

Quadriceps stretch – *Stand near a wall for support and bend your right leg behind you and grab your ankle on the back of your trainer. Gently pull your heel up and back until you feel a stretch in the front thigh. Keep the knees together and supporting leg a little soft. Hold for 15 seconds and change legs.*

Step 8
Chest Stretch – *With feet hip-width apart and legs slightly bent, clasp your hands behind your back and lift your arms behind you until you can feel the stretch across your chest. Hold for 15 seconds.*

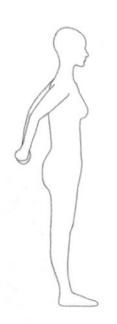

Main Workout
Do each of these strength-training moves once before moving on to the next exercise. Try to keep your rest time between exercises to a minimum. This will keep your heart rate up and maximise your calorie burn:

Press ups – (targets chest and arms)
Kneel down on the floor and place your hands shoulder width apart in front of you. Adjust your body position so that your knees are as far away from your hands as you can tolerate. Make sure your backside is tucked in and your tummy muscles are pulled in tight! With weight on hands, slowly lower yourself towards the floor, before pushing back up to the starting position. Aim to repeat this exercise 15–20 times.

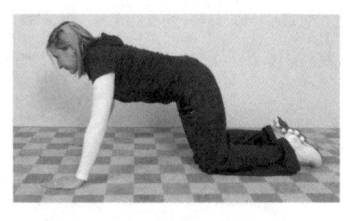

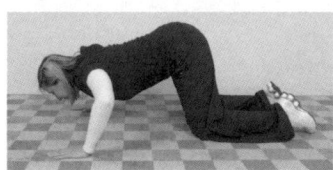

Squats – (targets thighs, hips and backside)

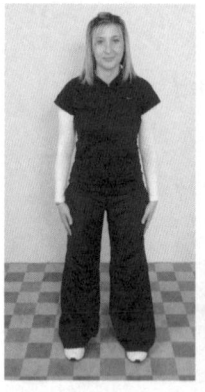

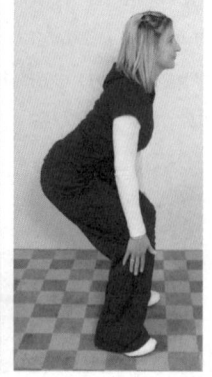

Taking care to keep your stomach pulled in tight and your bum tucked under.

Stand with your feet hip-width apart and knees slightly bent. Keep your back straight and hands on hips or out in front slightly clasped together. Bend your knees to about 90°, allowing your body to lean forwards slightly until at right angles to your thighs. Almost imagine there is a chair behind you and you're going to push your bum back as if to sit on it but instead you are just going to stand back up before your bum hits the seat. Aim for 15–20 repetitions. You could even use the water bottles or cans of beans to hold in each hand and hold your arms straight down either side of your leg.

FIT

Jumping Jacks (aerobic exercise, calorie burner)

This is a fabulous calorie burner. Starting in a normal standing position, with arms by sides, jump your feet apart and lift your arms into the air. As you jump your feet back together, bring your arms back down. Repeat as many times as you can and build up to doing them for a minute, putting as much energy into each 'jumping jack' as you can!

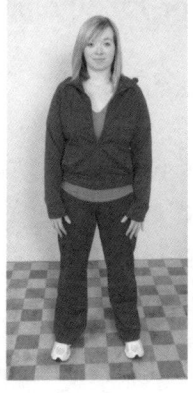

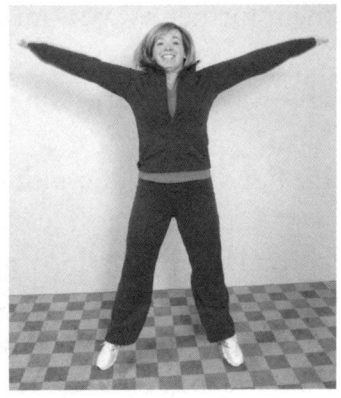

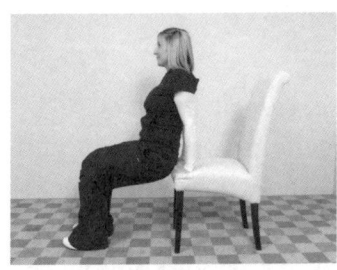

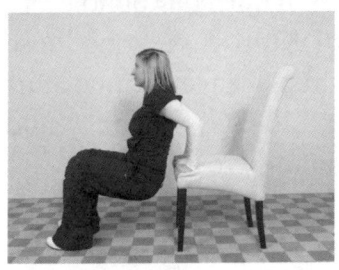

Dips – (targets backs of arms or BINGO WINGS!)

Sit on a sturdy chair and place hands either side of your hips with fingers pointing in the same direction as you are facing. Slowly lower yourself off the edge of the chair, bending from the elbow to support your body weight. Come down until your elbows are bent at right angles and then push yourself back up. Start

THE SLIM GIRL'S BOOK OF SECRETS

with feet fairly close to the chair and progress by taking them further away. Aim for 15–20 repetitions

Hip Raises – (targets backside and hips)
Lie flat on the floor with your knees bent and your feet close to your body. Drive your hips up into the air, focusing on using the muscles in your gluts (bum) to lift your body weight. Hold this for a second before lowering down to the floor. To progress, try lifting one leg into the air and focusing on each side individually. Aim for 15–20 repetitions.

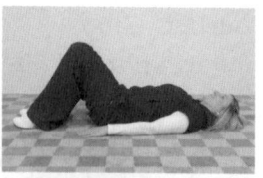

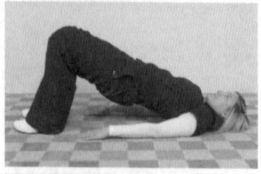

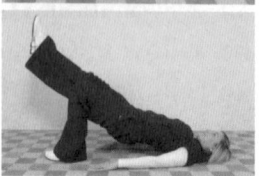

Jog on the Spot (aerobic exercise, calorie burner)

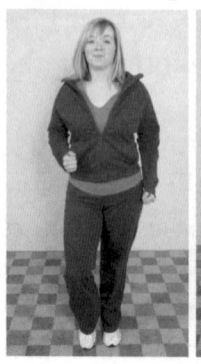

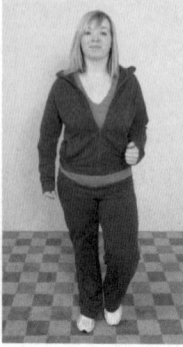

Revitalise your body with a quick jog. The quicker you jog, the more calories you'll burn but build up to it!! Keep your arms loose and place feet firmly. Start at 20–30 seconds and build up to a minute.

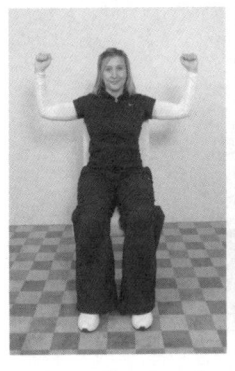

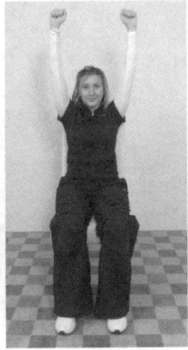

Shoulder Press (targets your shoulder muscles and upper arms.)

Sit on a chair with your feet flat on the floor. Hold a water bottle or can of something in each hand at shoulder height, elbows out and palms facing forward. Press the bottles or cans up and in, until your arms are almost straight, so they nearly touch above your head. Don't let them stray back and forth and then slowly lower to the starting position. Aim for 15–20 repetitions

Step Ups (targets your lower body muscles)

Use your stairs but please ensure the step isn't too high (one step or two) you shouldn't be lifting your knees higher than your hips.

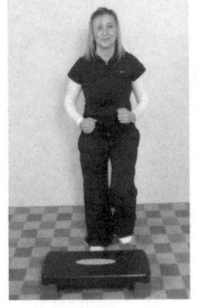

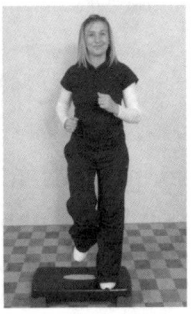

Stand facing your step. Step up with one foot, placing your whole foot flat on the step. Keep your back straight and your head and neck relaxed but in line with your torso. Step up with your other foot so that both feet are flat on the step. Step down one foot at a time. Aim for 10 step ups on each leg and try to increase to 15–20.

Skipping

Take yourself back to your playground days and imagine you are holding an imaginary skipping rope and just skip. Aim for 20 – 30 seconds to start and build up to minute.

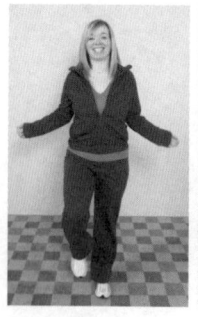

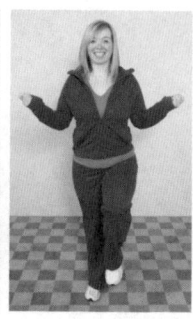

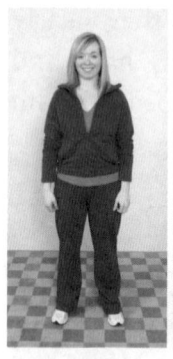

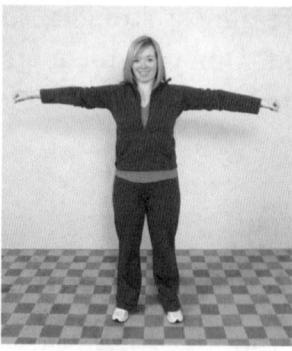

Lateral Raises

(works all three sections of your shoulder muscles) Stand with your feet hip-width apart, knees slightly bent. Hold a water bottle or can of soup/beans in each hand, starting with your arms by your side, palms facing inwards. Keep your abdominals tight.

Slowly lift your arms away from your sides, more or less straight but keeping your elbows slightly bent, until your hands are at shoulder level. Keep palms facing down your and return your arms to the start. Aim for 15–20 repetitions.

Superwoman – (targets core muscles and improves balance and co-ordination)

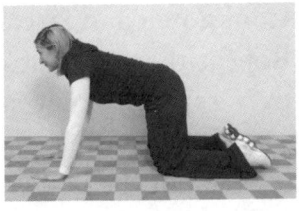

Kneel on all fours, making sure that hands are aligned with shoulders and knees are directly under hips. Elevate your right arm and your right leg simultaneously, extending the limbs fully and keeping your back as flat as you can. Aim to create as much length through your body as you can, reaching your hand forward and stretching your toes back. Slowly lower and switch sides. Do 10 repetitions on each side.

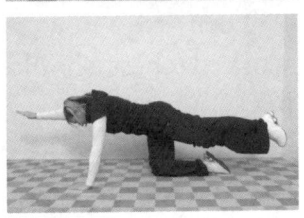

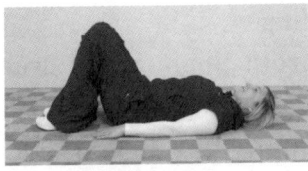

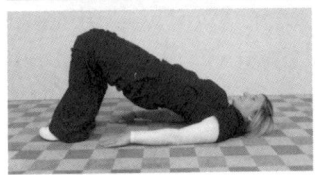

Pelvic Lifts

Same as hip raises but emphasises working on the transverse abdominus muscles which is the set of muscles that resemble a big girdle and sit underneath your superficial tummy muscles. Lie flat on your back, knees bent and feet flat on the floor. Lift your hips towards the ceiling until they are parallel with your knees and hold this position for 10 seconds and then lower your bum back down towards the floor. Repeat 5 times.

Cool-down and Stretch

Repeat the warm up but gradually reduce the intensity over several minutes. Then lie flat on your back and stretch your arms over your head and point the toes to stretch out the body.

Then do a few stretches of all the major muscles worked (chest, shoulders, front and back thigh and lower back.)

Hamstring: Lying on your back, bend both knees and feet flat on the floor. Take one leg up and with both hands support the leg either at the back of the thigh or calf. Gently straighten the leg until you feel a stretch at the back of your leg. Hold for 15–30 seconds. Then repeat with other leg.

Bringing yourself slowly to standing ...

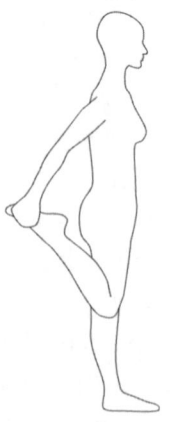

Quad stretch/front thigh: Stand near a wall for support and bend your left leg behind you and grab your ankle or the back of your trainer. Gently pull your heel up and back until you feel a stretch in the front of your thigh. Keep the knees together and the supporting leg a little soft. Hold for 15 seconds and change legs.

Chest Stretch: With feet hip-width apart and legs slightly bent, clasp your hands behind your back and lift your arms behind you until you can feel the stretch across your chest. Hold for 15 seconds.

Shoulder Stretch: Stand as above; take your right arm across your body so your forearm is by your left shoulder. Place your left hand on your upper arm to stretch a bit further. Hold for 10 seconds and then swap arms.

To start with, the warm up and cool-down and the circuit of exercises once through may only take 15–20 minutes but as you get fitter or if you feel more able you can try doing the main circuit of exercises twice through and then as you progress take it up to 3 times. You be the judge, obviously this will increase the duration and intensity of your workout.

Weekly Plans and Progressions

Now that all the routines are explained I just want to run through the first 5 weeks and how you can progress things a little each week or as you feel ready. The plan is so flexible that you can adapt it to suit your needs and you can progress, as and when you feel ready. Once you have completed the plan you can start over again and simply increase the intensity by yourself or log on anytime at **www.slimgirlsboxofsecrets.com** for the latest moves and a little dose of motivation from Alba and me.

Week 1

Start with doing the sculpt and blast routine twice a week. This is a perfect way to introduce exercise into your life at 20–30 minutes per session. It will start to gently introduce your muscles to the wonderful world of exercise. Go by how you feel and by how much time you can allocate to the workout. Remember, even if you do 2 lots of 15 minutes – one at the start of the day and one at the end – instead of the full 30 minutes this will be better than not doing it at all. Remember little and often!!!

If you can only do the workout once to start with that's still fantastic. Build yourself up – this way you will ensure that you stay motivated and will be more likely to keep it up rather than want to stop because it's too difficult. This is about making it as easy as you like.

If you can, add in a cardio exercise session. You could go for a brisk/power walk, swim or gentle cycle – whatever you enjoy the most and feel like doing.

You can even keep doing week 1 for 2 weeks and then progress. You don't have to do the workouts on the exact days that are on the plan – fit it into your week however it works best for you. Just ensure you don't do the workouts back to back. Try to leave a day's rest so that you give your muscles time to rest and repair (this is when the magic will happen, so rest is a must!)

Week 2
Keep things as in Week 1. Two sculpt and blast workouts (you can find this on the accompanying DVD) and one cardio exercise. If you feel ready, you can increase the intensity of the workouts by repeating the circuit in the sculpt and blast workout 2 or 3 times or by adding an extra 5 minutes onto your cardio workout.

Week 3
Try 2 sculpt and blasts and 2 cardio workouts.

Week 4
By now, you will be really starting to feel the benefits. You will be feeling more energetic and, as long as you have been following a healthy eating plan, your clothes will be feeling looser and your body internally will be benefiting from the changes. In this week you can start to progress things a little more and start to challenge yourself a little more (but only if you feel ready). Still do the same weekly routine as Week 3, but you have the option to increase your effort levels in the workouts and increase the workout time of your cardio session. Another suggestion would be to add some new exercises into your sculpt and blast routine (see below). Go to the pick and mix section of your DVD to see these moves.

PICK AND MIX EXERCISES – to choose from when you're ready for a little more of a challenge

Wide Leg Squats

This works the front and back of your thighs and your bottom and lower back.

From the basic squat position, take your feet out approximately half as much again and turn your toes out. Imagine a clock face – your left foot is pointing to 10 and right to 2. Now tip your hips back, keep the chest up and looking straight ahead sink the hips back until your thighs are parallel with the floor. Ensure your knees are in line with your feet (10 to 2). You can progress this even more by holding a big water bottle in front of you, making sure that you don't let the weight pull you forward, keep your shoulder squeezed back and keep your chest high. Aim for 15–20 repetitions.

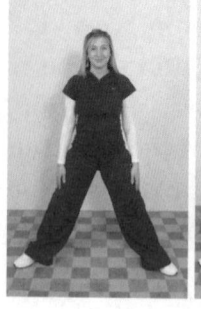

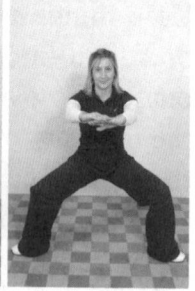

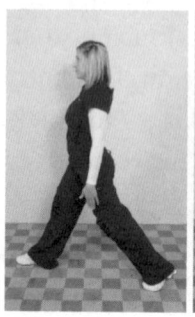

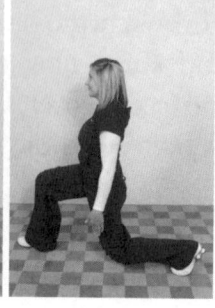

Lunges

Place one-foot forward about one stride-length from the back leg. Keep your hips facing straight ahead and arms by your side; lift your back heel of your back leg. Keep your abdominals pulled in – as always and body upright. Then bend your knees to bring your front knee over your front foot and the back knee should bend to a 90° angle, then drive back up off both your front foot and toes on the back leg – all the time maintain your body in an upright position. Aim for 15–20 on each leg.

The Plank
This does not involve finding a pirate ship and a parrot. ☺
Works the stomach and deep core muscles
Lie face down on the floor
Bring your elbows in and underneath your shoulders with your palms down.

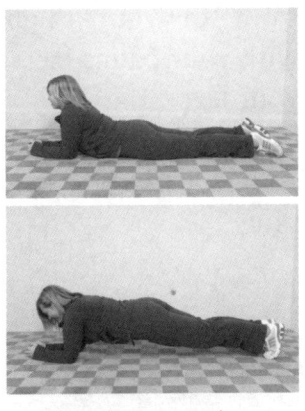

Breathe out as you draw your stomach in and raise your hips from the floor, keeping your shoulders and back in the same position. Aim to hold for as long as you can, build up to a minute or more if you can.

A few quick safety tips for the plank:
Don't hunch your shoulders or raise your bum too high or let it sink, keep your body in a straight line and pull in through your stomach and keep breathing.

To work up to this you can start by doing the half plank, which is keeping your lower legs and feet on the floor and raising up on to your knees so only your thighs are off the floor and maintaining a straight line from your knees to your head.

Upright Row
Stand with your feet hip width apart and knees slightly bent. Hold a water bottle or can in each hand in front of your thighs with your palms facing your legs.

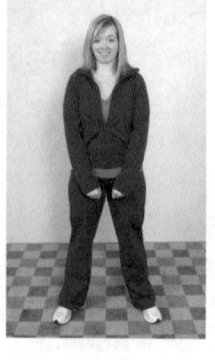

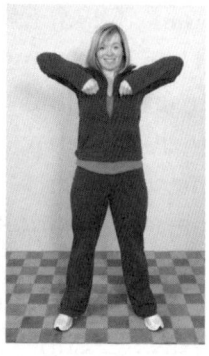

Slowly raise the bottles to chin height, keeping your palms facing towards your body. Aim for 15–20 repetitions.

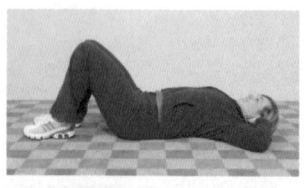

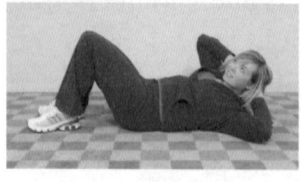

Oblique Crunch
Lie on your back with your knees together and legs raised so that your thighs are at 90° to the floor. Keep your tummy muscles pulled in tight and your back pressed into the floor. Place your hands by your ears. Raise one elbow and shoulder towards your opposite knee. Return to the start. Do the next oblique with your other elbow and then alternate sides until you've completed the reps. Aim for 15–20 repetitions.

Jump Squats

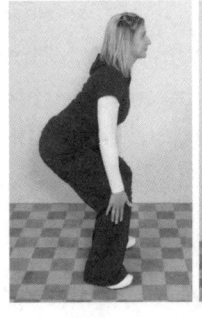

Start in a squat position, feet hip width apart and hips lowered, bound into the air pushing upwards, landing in the same position you started in. Repeat, making sure to land with knees bent to reduce impact on your knees. This is an intense, fat burning exercise. Aim for 10 'jump squats'!

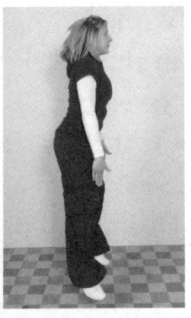

Pec Dec

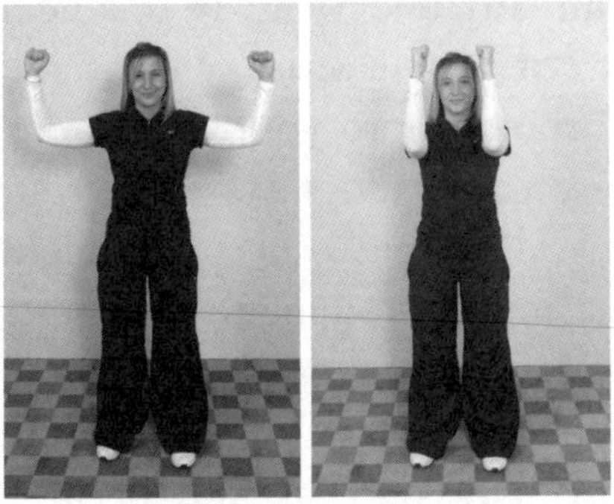

Stand with your feet hip width apart, with a bottle or can in each hand, take your arms out to the sides at shoulder level, bend your arms so there is a 90° bend at the elbows and palms facing out, and knuckles towards the ceiling. Then bring your arms across the front of your body, so your elbows meet, keeping the bend in the elbows and squeeze through your chest muscles to bring elbows together. Aim for 15–20 repetitions.

Week 5

In this Week you'll be feeling your fitness levels starting to really pick up and therefore will be ready to really go for it in each workout. The workouts stay the same as Week 4 but again try to take the challenge a little further. Do the sculpt and circuit 3 – 4 times if you can or try to advance the moves in the routine. Go for a little longer in your cardio workouts, always ensuring you judge it by how you're feeling. Keep up the good work, we'll be seeing a lot less of you very soon.

Fun Food Facts

With your exercise plan already underway, in this next section I'm going to share with you a series of ideas and principles for you to incorporate into your day to day eating habits. Some of these you'll adopt as part of your life, some you'll do when you can and others you might reject altogether. The most important thing to remember is that this is not a diet because diets alone don't work in the long-term. The yo-yo effect on your weight as a result of dieting puts a tremendous stress on your body, because when it comes to nutrition your body thrives on regularity, it is far better to simply eat more efficiently on a regular basis, than to eat poorly and then starve yourself. The following 6 principles are small, simple adjustments you can make to the way you eat. Over time, along with regular exercise they will have a marked positive effect on your body (inside and out!!). I have chosen these specific ideas to give you more energy and ensure that you get the biggest benefit from the effort you're putting.

SUGGESTION 1: Minimise intake of simple carbohydrates.

Eating sugar and white flour products such as white bread, cereals, white rice, white pasta, chocolate, confectionery, alcohol and sugary drinks will cause your blood – glucose levels to fluctuate causing highs and lows in energy levels. When you hit an energy low you are more likely to reach for a quick fix high sugar snack which will ultimately resulting in weight gain. Not too clever!

SUGGESTION 2: Always try to eat breakfast.

Breakfast is essential, it gives you the fuel to help sustain your energy levels and kick start your metabolism for the day. It can be hard to fit in breakfast if you have a busy lifestyle but making a little time for it is so important when controlling your weight in the long term. I know some people say they just can't face breakfast in the morning – in this case a fruit smoothie would be a good option. You can even get them with your skinny latté in the coffee shop now, how cool is that?

SUGGESTION 3: Eat little and often.

Eating the right foods little and often is vital as this gives you a constant supply of energy throughout the day and avoids your blood sugar levels dropping which causes hunger, tiredness and emotional food cravings.

SUGGESTION 4: Eat fibre rich foods.

There are many benefits in eating fibre. It's not a nutrient but is extremely healthy and can improve digestion, reduce levels of harmful cholesterol, reduce your risk of heart attacks and stroke, help control your blood-sugar levels and fill you up, helping you to maintain or lose weight. You can get fibre from whole grains, vegetables, fruit, beans, lentils and oats.

SUGGESTION 5: Drink fresh juice

Most people do not eat enough fresh fruit and vegetables on a daily basis. Freshly squeezed juices are a quick and enjoyable way of getting the vitamins and minerals necessary to maintain healthy living. The vitamins and minerals from freshly squeezed juices are absorbed into the body within minutes of consumption. Fruit and vegetables eaten in a normal manner can take up to 6 hours to digest in which time a considerable proportion is by-passed as waste. Health professionals recommend that a daily intake of Vitamin C should be 60mg – 1/2 pint of freshly squeezed orange juice contains 100mg. If you can make the time to clean it buy a juicer and juice your own fruit and veg.

Ali's Top Tip – The problem I've always had with juicing is that no matter which machine you buy (and I've tried lots) cleaning it always takes far longer than the juicing. So here's my top tip for helping you find time to juice.

You know when you go to the supermarket and put your fruit and veg in those really thin plastic bags? Well, they make great liners for the pulp hopper of your juicer, they are just about the right size and mean that all the pulp is collected neatly, ready to be thrown away. Genius! And makes me feel better about using the plastic too.

Here are just a few of the benefits fresh juices can offer you:

- Helps combat colds and flu
- Helps keep skin looking healthy and vibrant
- Keeps gums strong and healthy
- Improves your memory (what does..?)
- Helps prevent migraines
- Speeds up the natural healing process
- Increase resistance to heart disease by improving cholesterol levels
- Relieves allergies, eczema, sinusitis and asthma
- Helps regulate blood pressure, heartbeat, nerve and muscle functions

Fresh juices are packed with nutrients, they increase our vitality, improve our physique, help us ward off disease and put less strain on our digestive system. Go on get juicing!

SUGGESTION 6: Follow the 80:20 rule
This means try and eat healthily 80% of the time, 20% of the time you can stray and have a few treats without feeling guilty – this stops the boredom and frustration associated with normal diet regimes.

You have now reached the end of the fitness part – Phew! You have already made the biggest step by reading this section and possibly even trying the DVD and the exercises – you are well on your way!! Remember, the first workout will always seem the most challenging but the more you practice the more you will become comfortable and familiar with the exercises. Soon you will be feeling amazing and looking at a new you in the mirror and getting that new shape will not have felt like a chore or struggle at all! ☺

If you do think that it's too easy, please go with it anyway. Success is a process not a one off hard workout. The key is little and often but please do push yourself a bit harder if that's more satisfying for you.

Healthy

You'll be familiar with the phrase Fit AND Healthy. I used to think they were one and the same thing, a bit like Country AND Western.

I have no idea what the textbook difference is or even if there is one but here is my take on the difference between Fitness and Healthiness.

By health I really mean happy and balanced and centred whichever way you think about yourself when you are living as the authentic you. That is health to me. The next section is about you and that feeling of living your values. Keep getting slimmer and fitter but next up is Life Balance …

Happiness and freedom begin with a clear understanding of one principle – some things are within your control and some things are not.

Epictetus (circa 100 AD)

There is another old saying, simply 'healthy mind, healthy body'. In this section we are going to look at what could be called 'healthy, life balance'. Now you're getting slimmer and have learned some of the simple secrets of being slim, now you are exercising and getting fitter, it follows that the next step on your journey will be getting and maintaining a healthy balance in the rest of your life.

Quick question! What stops you from living a happy, healthy and balanced life? Take a moment and just jot down the first 5 things that come to mind. You can do it here or in your journal.

HEALTHY

1. _____
2. _____
3. _____
4. _____
5. _____

Now have a look through your answers and notice which ones are outside your control … and which ones you have made up and which ones are not real. It's an interesting exercise. I used to find that lots of the stress in my life came from trying to control things that were outside my control anyway … Let me explain.

My friend and mentor *Michael Neill* first got me thinking about this when I was complaining that some things weren't going the way I wanted them to go. We were having an interesting conversation about the things I could control and those I couldn't. That is, those that I could directly or indirectly influence in some way and those things I could do absolutely nothing about. We decided that there were 3 main groupings but only 2 worth speaking about. Those I could control and by that I mean I can make happen reliably at will and those that I may be able to 'influence' in some way. There is obviously a third group of things I have absolutely no control over whatsoever.

My life is not the same as yours but I'll share what I learned with you anyway.

I can absolutely reliably control ...
What I do or don't do in any given moment
What I say or don't say at any given time
What I choose to focus my attention on
What I choose to make important
What I welcome into my life and what I reject

I can influence ...
How I feel most of the time
Other people some of the time
The physical environment around me
The economy, to varying degrees (I can spend or save or donate or receive)
My weight
The way I look and feel

I can't control ...
How I feel at any given moment
What thoughts pass through my mind
What happens to me next
What other people think, do or say
What happens in the wider world

What I found so interesting in this little exploration was just how *little* we directly control (essentially it's only our attitude, words, choices and actions) but how *much* we can directly influence from our inner environment to the people around us.

In Michael's book *Feel Happy Now!*, he shares the following story:

While interviewing Olympic rowers at the 1996 Olympics, sports broadcaster Charlie Jones spoke with a number of the competing athletes. Any time he asked them a question about something which was outside their control (like the weather, the strengths and weaknesses of their opponents or what might go wrong during a race), the Olympians would respond with the phrase 'That's outside my boat.'

By refusing to focus on anything which was beyond their control, these athletic champions were able to bring all their resources to bear on what was within their control – everything from their physiology, mental maps and story to the actions that they took preparing for and competing in the actual event."

In my own life, I've found that focusing exclusively on what's 'in my boat' not only increases my effectiveness but reduces my stress level dramatically. Logically it makes sense but how often do you find yourself getting frustrated and trying to control something that's outside your control anyway?

As the baseball player Mickey Rivers once said:

I'm not going to worry about the things I can't control, because if I can't control them there's no point in worrying about them; and I'm not going to worry about the things I can control, because if I can control them there's no point in worrying about them.

What's in your boat?
1. Pick a time from the past when you were feeling stressed or anxious.
2. Have a careful think about it and notice what it is that was the source of the stress.
3. Is it something that you can control?
4. If it wasn't and I'm fairly sure it wasn't, what parts of the situation could you positively influence?

Play the "Can Control/Can Influence/Can't Control" game. For every item you come up with that you don't control, write down what you do control that will positively influence the result you would like to achieve. For example:

I don't control my weight but I do control what I put in my mouth and how much exercise I do.

Or

I was at an outdoor music event this weekend here in Scotland and found myself worrying about the weather and how it would dampen our spirits and fun. Obviously I don't control the weather but I do control the packing of my wellies, waterproofs and midge repellent (ah, the Scottish summer) and can influence the mood and attitude of my friends by keeping my own spirits high. I'm pleased to say we're all home in one piece, nobody drowned in the mud and we had a great time, despite the elements conspiring against us.

So, back to you, take the "control" challenge. Focus on what is within your control or influence and notice what happens.

You can keep a log in your journal. If you find yourself spending time "outside your boat", just climb back in, dry yourself off and keep paddling!

Letting go of struggle

When I first began to explore the idea of letting go of struggle it felt a little alien to me. The person I was working with was trying to convince me that I could have what I wanted without having to struggle for it. Now that went against my entire child hood upbringing. 'If something's worth having, it's worth working for right?' Of course you need to struggle – what's the alternative? Just wishing your life away?

Well, actually I was wrong, as I have been many times! You see, my journey to this point has been a very personal one. These are not just regurgitated theories I've picked up from self-help books over the years. These are the techniques that I have found really work for me and with my clients. You don't have to struggle but at first it can feel a little weird to let go of it.

What are you struggling with right now? Are you prepared to let go of that struggle or are you so attached to it that struggling almost feels comfortable to you? We are conditioned that struggle is almost to be expected. Only the other day I received an email from a client asking me for help in her 'fight' with her weight. Why does it have to be a 'fight'. I know, we are 'supposed' to 'try'

THE SLIM GIRL'S BOOK OF SECRETS

to succeed against the odds, to strive and graft and if we're lucky we might be rewarded but it doesn't have to be like that.

I'm going to ask you a very straight question.

Are you ready to give up on 'your struggle'? You will be surprised how many people aren't. What would you do if you didn't have to struggle? Let's do a quick exercise. I'd like you to close your eyes and think about something you're currently struggling with. Where do you feel that sense of struggle? How do you carry that around with you? Where do you feel that in your body? Does it feel light or heavy? Does it feel like it's moving or still? Just note your instinctive responses.

Now I'd like you to think about what it would be like to let go of this feeling. How do you feel about that? Does it feel like it will be a relief to get rid of it or does that thought actually feel like a bit of a struggle in itself? Does the idea of ridding yourself of that feeling of struggle feel like you are losing a part of you? Does a part of you feel like it has always been there? So, let me ask you again, how do you feel about giving up on struggle and just allowing things to be easier? By holding onto the idea that it has to be difficult, you are putting an artificial barrier between you and your happiness.

What do you struggle with? _____

Do you feel attached to it? _____

Are you ready to let go of that struggle now? This might be an obvious 'yes' but I really want you to think about whether you are really ready to give up on the things you've been struggling with for good.

8 | DIFY – Letting go of struggle

If you are, then let it go now ... Listen to the "letting go of struggle" track on your CD and get ready to move forward with ease like never before.

If you're not quite ready yet, think about what would have to happen in order for you to let it go. And then think about what you can do to bring that about... In the easiest way possible, of course.

Are you ready to do that? If yes then you are ready to give up on the struggle now ... Listen to the track and let's move on.

Self sabotage –

Do you ever find yourself sabotaging all your good work and not really understanding why? I know people who do this in every area of their life but one thing is constant: people tend to sabotage the thing that they want most in life. I know people who crave being in a loving balanced relationship yet sabotage things with every romantic liaison just to prove themselves right, that they can never have what they want. Just the same, I know people who sabotage themselves with food, with alcohol, with drugs, in fact with just about anything that can be damaging.

There are many stories of athletes sabotaging themselves so that they don't have to win and so they can keep telling their story. We all have a story about who we are and how we have come to be where we are. Whatever your story, I'm sure you've told it many times to yourself and to others and that, by now, it feels very real. One of the best pieces of advice I was ever given was 'stop telling your story and start living your life.' Good advice. Your story is usually made up of the 'reasons' why things are the way they are and therefore they are fixed that way. That's just the way it is. Well it's not, it can be any way you want it to be but first you have to stop telling the story that is holding you in the place you're in.

One of the reasons that many talking therapies don't work is that describing and re-telling your story doesn't make it go away. In fact, quite the opposite is true. As with anything, the more you practice the better you get.

Please stop telling your story and get on with writing the next chapter of your life. From today you have a blank page and with my help a sharper pencil. You cannot change the past but you can seriously influence the future. So let's get on with it.

I was attending a conference in the Virgin Islands last year when I met a performance coach who shared the story of one of the world's leading golfers. He explained that many times she would be leading tournaments with a few holes to play but somehow she would find a way to finish second or third. In fact, she managed to do that many times in a row. There appeared to be no reason for it, she just lost form with a few holes to go. When it came down to it, she just wouldn't win. Well, that's until they started to do a little bit of digging and uncovered the real reason for her self sabotage. You see it emerged that she actually had a fear of public speaking …

She had a fear of public speaking because she didn't like the way she looked or sounded on screen and so her subconscious found a way to prevent her from having to make a victory speech by making sure she missed a few putts or put a couple of drives in the rough. Yes, your subconscious is that clever and powerful!

Can you see now why it's so important to get your subconscious working with you? It's always on your side but sometimes it's not fully aligned with your goals.

I was working with a client recently, (I'll call her Angelina to protect her identity and because it'll make her smile if she reads this) doing a weight loss session. The session began in the usual kind of way. She was telling me how she really, really wanted to lose weight but no matter how hard she tried she would somehow find herself reaching for the fridge and before she knew it the cheese cake that she didn't even want would be just a distant and much regretted memory. 'I just don't understand it, I really want to lose weight but something just takes over and I have to eat it, even though I know I don't want it and know that I'll feel terrible and guilty about it afterwards.' Now, I've done this a few times so had a fair idea of the key question, the one that would unlock her hidden positive intention and ultimately set her free. You can try this for yourself right now … What are you afraid would happen if you lost weight? Or to put it another way, what does being overweight protect you from? ... Think about it carefully. *I've included that actual conversation here as I really think it'll help you.*

Angelina thought for a while then said, 'Well, if I lost weight I'd probably find myself in a relationship'

Ali: Ok, good – why's that a bad thing?
Angelina: Well because then I'd get hurt.
Ali: What else could it be?
Angelina: If I lost weight I'd probably have the confidence to do lots of the things I make excuses for not being able to do
Ali: Why's that bad?
Angelina: Because I'm not sure I'd actually be able to do them and then I'd be disappointed, it's better not to know
Ali: What else could it be?
Angelina: Actually now that I think about it, I guess if I'm overweight and the world is hard on me then I have a reason, if I'm slim and things don't go my way then I must be about me and I'm not sure I can handle that. It's like if I'm fat and the world hates me then it must be because I'm fat, but if I'm not fat and the world still hates me, then it must be me.?
Ali: Hmmm ...
Angelina: No way, I'm actually hiding behind being over weight, wow I've never thought of it like that before.
Ali: And can you now see why your subconscious would try to keep you overweight? If, on one hand we have

hurt, disappointment, rejection and pain, and on the other hand we have cheesecake, I'd choose the cheese cake too!

Angelina: Wow – that totally makes sense, so how do I change that?

Ali: That's the easy bit, even just by realising that this is what's happening helps to break its spell but we'll use some hypnotherapy and an NLP technique called a 6-step reframe to sort it out.

(The same techniques are on your The Slim Girl's Key Secret CD, you might like to listen to it when you get to the end of this section, or a little later when it's more convenient and then as often as you like.)

Your subconscious always wants what's best for you and in her case it was protecting her from pain and disappointment. Clever eh? But not really very useful when your goal is to win golf tournaments or losing weight or being more confident.

So … what might your subconscious be doing for you that is actually holding you back? What is it that stops you from letting go of your limiting beliefs and just going for it?

You'll not be surprised to learn that once the fear of public speaking was sorted out using some of the techniques you have here and her conscious goals and her sub-conscious were aligned Annika Sorenstam won almost everything in sight and went all the way to No. 1 in the world.

This quote is included with Angelina's kind permission.

"*Ali helped me to realise that the negative attitudes I was feeding myself were the true source of my weight gain.*
I find it impossible to sum up the effect this has had on me because with my mind now working for me rather than against me I feel there is no limit to what I can achieve."

If it were true of one of the world's best golfers, what makes you think you'd be any different? You're not. I'm not. We all have stuff that holds us back and stops us from living the lives we want.

I know that in my own life I noticed that sometimes when I had a big meeting to prepare for or an important email to send, I would tend to put it off and put it off and put it off. Now, these were meetings that would undoubtedly help me to make my dreams come a bit closer. So why did I leave it to the last minute? Simple. At some level, I had a fear of making my life better; a fear of change or a fear of what it would mean if I gave up on my old ways and stepped up to the mark. Happily, I've got over it now and love the challenge of being creative and welcoming new things into my life, but you can be sure that the only real thing stopping me for so long was me and it wasn't really real after all, it was just a thought. Sure, I told myself stories about why I couldn't do it or why it was the way it was but the truth is that it was the way it was because I made it that way. Consciously or sub-consciously I made it that way and you do too. Until now that is ... You have the chance right now to (best Michael Caine voice) 'blow the bloody doors off' your limiting beliefs and step into the real you.

So here's a thought ... We spoke earlier about letting go of the connection between thoughts and actions, I hope you're getting on well with that by now? Let me expand this idea a bit further for you. The idea comes from the principles of 'Psychology of Mind' formed by a fellow Scot, Syd Banks and then further developed by George and Jack Pransky. As an aside, if you are having difficulties in your relationships or know someone who is, check out *The Relationship Handbook* by *George Pransky*. It's a wonderful new way of looking at and interacting with your life and those who are in it. Anyway back to the point, we are all born, happy, healthy and content but, over time, we get stretched and pulled by who we think we 'should' be, what we think we 'should' be doing and pulled this way and that by events in our lives.

I'd like you to imagine a large spring, you know the kind you used to play with as a child. In its natural state, it's relaxed and quite content to just happily sit, full of coiled energy but happy just to be still.

However, we tend to allow ourselves to get stretched out of shape, to get pulled in different directions. The more we get pulled out of shape, the more tension and stress we feel in our lives. All the time all our spring wants to do is to return to its natural state of being: relaxed, content, loving and just, well, happy.

When a spring is stretched and under strain you don't have to push it back into shape, you don't have to force it or struggle to get it back to normal, it doesn't take years of therapy, it just has an innate memory of who it is and what it looks like and naturally wants to get back to that state. All you have to do is let go.

Let go of whatever is keeping it stressed, whatever it is that's stopping it from being the way it is supposed to be and it will find its way back effortlessly and quicker than you think.

The point, in case you have missed it, is that YOU are that spring, YOU are an innately happy and health person but you have got stretched out of shape and the stress in your life comes from your innate desire to return to the way you're supposed to be.

It makes sense when you think about it but I'll concede that for me it was a whole new way of looking at life. Starting from a place where everything is ok, you can just let it be the way you should be, it can be as easy as that.

9 | DIFY – What pulls you out of shape?

So, if you're with me so far, then let's take this idea a step further ... What is it that pulls you out of shape? What is it that causes tension in your spring? Quickly make a list of some of the things that cause you to be tense and

HEALTHY

stressed and stop you from being the healthy, happy person you are supposed to be?

1. _____
2. _____
3. _____
4. _____
5. _____

Now obviously I can't see your answers but I'll bet you a cup of coffee (you can claim it later) that most of the items on your list are 'things', stuff on the outside of you. When I first did this exercise my answers looked something like this.

1. The location I live in
2. My relationship with my partner
3. My burning desire to be successful
4. My knee injury which 10 years on still gives me pain
5. The thought that maybe I'm not good enough

I'm sure these are not the same as yours but I'll bet there are some similarities. It was in the last answer that I realised what had actually been keeping me in the place I was in.

Conventional positive thinking theory would probably have said some variation on 'replace that negative thought with a positive one' e.g. 'maybe I'm not good enough – NO, I AM GREAT!" or the NLP version' take that negative thought and turn the voice all the way down' or the coaching version 'what actions could you take to make yourself better?' All very valid ways of dealing with it, but the secret is bigger and simpler than that and I'm going to share it with you now. If you get nothing else from this book, apart from a slimmer waistline, then this is worth the cover price alone …

The distinction is simple. All of my answers, all of the things that were stopping me from being the ME that I 'should' be were just thoughts. Just thoughts! It was my thoughts that were holding me in that place and preventing me from springing back to the real me. Let me show the sub text to that same list again

1. The location I live in – that where I live matters; that where I live says something negative about me; that I 'should' be living somewhere else; that I was unhappy 'because' of this.
2. My relationship with my partner – that she doesn't 'get' me; that I'm not worthy of being with someone so wonderful.
3. My burning desire to be successful – that I will be successful once I have 'achieved' something; that success is a 'something'; that I'm not already successful; that I will gain something (happiness) from this 'success'.
4. My knee injury which, 10 years on, still gives me pain – that I am hard done by; that I'm unlucky; that I have a valid reason to not exercise; that I have a good hard luck or 'if only' story to tell.

5. Maybe I'm not good enough – not good enough for what? that there is a point you can reach that is 'good enough'; that not feeling satisfied with my skill level at this stage is a bad thing; that my self worth is measured by my knowledge and skill level.

These are really the thoughts that lurk behind the statements. Can you make the distinction that all of those 'could' be real if I chose to make them real or all of those could just as easily be 'just thoughts' that can pass in a second and never bother me again.

If I gave power to any one of those thoughts, I could feel very down and despondent, or not, but that's my choice. Thoughts appear very real and we can make them real by giving them power and taking actions based on them but the thought itself is just that – Just a thought.

Re-visit your list and add all the thoughts and assumptions that are behind the answers on your list. Notice what they are and then for each in turn jot down if it's really real or just a thought. Now I'll bet you a refill that your list looks quite different from before.

Don't put up with it!

Which thoughts are you making real and then tolerating?

It reminds me of a story about boiling a frog. It's a well known fable which I have been unable to accurately reference to its source, but I first heard it from a friend when I was unhappy in a situation many years ago. I'm

THE SLIM GIRL'S BOOK OF SECRETS

not suggesting that you do this (although there are many listings on the internet as to whether this story would actually work in practice). Please be nice to our amphibian friends ...

If you drop a frog into boiling water it will instinctively jump straight back out ... (Phew! No point in trying it). However, if you place a frog in a pan of cold water, then gradually turn up the heat, the frog will at first get comfortably warm, then cosy, then accept that it's getting a little hot in here but quite happily sit there and boil to death. This is also true of people. I'm sure you have been in situations where you have gradually adjusted to accept things over time, a little at a time till you find things heating up and find yourself in a place that you never thought you would be in and can't quite figure out how you got there. If you were dropped into that situation from scratch, you know you would jump straight back out ... and quick!

What are you tolerating in your life? What has the heat gradually got turned up on? What would you like to jump straight out of now?

Make a list of the top 5 things you put up with ...

1. _____
2. _____
3. _____
4. _____
5. _____

HEALTHY

Now -Take the same list and ask yourself 'what specifically is it about this situation that makes me wish I could jump back out?'

1. _____
2. _____
3. _____
4. _____
5. _____

What stops you?

1. _____
2. _____
3. _____
4. _____
5. _____

10 – DIFY – Just quit for the day

I remember when I was a student I had a series of temp jobs to help me pay my way. I hated every one of them but grudgingly did them dutifully as the cash came in handy. The best feeling I can remember from that time was on the days I just quit.

I remember one particular job that I quit 'because it was sunny'. Ok, I didn't really quit because it was sunny. I quit because it was a terrible job and the canned traditional Scottish music was driving me mad. But, one day I woke up, the sun was shining (that doesn't happen much in Scotland) and I just couldn't face 8 hours working inside a woollen mill. So I quit. I didn't call in sick, I just quit. I have never felt such relief, It was actually only when I quit that I realised just how much I hated it. I'm sure something similar has happened to you. Do you remember the feeling of relief at knowing that you didn't ever have to do that thing ever again? It might be your last day at school, it might be the day you left your old job or broke up from a bad relationship. It can feel so good to just know that you don't have to do it anymore.

Now, I feel I should point out here that I am not a quitter. I will stick at things and see them through with the best of them, but I have learned this cool little technique to keep me sane and get a sense of perspective on situations that I'm not happy in or sure about.

When I find myself in a situation I'm not happy with I just quit! For an hour or for the day or for as long as I need. You can always take the job back tomorrow or as soon as you're ready. But for today just quit! You'll get an amazing sense of relief at how good that feels, when you're able to get out of the heat and get a different perspective. If you're up to your neck in it, chances are if you're feeling bad you'll be making bad decisions any way. Feelings are our body's way of allowing us to gauge the quality of our thinking.

Bad feelings = bad thinking
So take the chance and – Quit!

HEALTHY

Pick something where you feel out of your depth in hot water.

Write it down here _____

Now, just take a moment to write your resignation from that situation right now.

I (*your name*) ....

hereby 'QUIT' from

.... for today

Signed ....

It's only from the outside that you can see clearly. It's only once you are out of the situation that you can see it for what it is, good or bad.

Imagine yourself as an artist painting on the canvas of your life. Sometimes it's a good idea to step back and get a sense of perspective on what you've been creating. That way when you go back to paint again you'll know what still needs attention. To put it simply.

Analyse from the outside–in then change from the inside-out.

Thinking about things differently now? What is the simplest thing that is 'in your boat' that you can change easily for each of the things you've been putting up with?

1. _____
2. _____
3. _____
4. _____
5. _____

When are you planning to do that?

1. _____
2. _____
3. _____
4. _____
5. _____

Now just go back through that list and note which of those are 'real' and which are really just 'thoughts' and we know that thoughts are not us and therefore not real, and therefore don't have to affect us at all.

Let me tell you a little story. Go and make yourself a low fat cocoa and, once you're sitting comfortably, then I'll begin.

It's a story about a little girl, we'll call her Emily. Now Emily was old enough to make some big decisions for herself and was curious to discover and explore the world that she lived in. Emily was a normal little girl in every way; she even had an imaginary friend called Thought. Thought and Emily went everywhere together, like hand in glove they were inseparable. Emily relied on Thought a lot and Thought relished the role and gave Emily answers and meaning whenever she needed them.

HEALTHY

Thought effortlessly guided Emily and sometimes, when she really needed it, Thought took over and just plain told Emily what to do.

Thought was so 'good' at running Emily's life that she took her friend's advice willingly – she never questioned it and the more she trusted Thought, the more she came to know that Thought was wise and wonderful and knew best and, well, Thought was always right. 'Thought really is such a good friend'.

Even though Emily had such a good friend, she wasn't a happy girl. Even though she knew that her voice within was there for her, she still managed to feel bad. She still managed to get upset and to feel a little lost sometimes. Because Thought was such a good friend Thought joined her when she was feeling bad, Thought was right there with her so that Emily could feel bad and have bad thoughts all at the same time. How good a friend is that?

Thought always matched Emily perfectly; Thought never got it wrong; Thought was never accidentally good when Emily was feeling bad; Thought was always right there with her. It felt comfortable for Emily. When she was feeling bad, the feeling was not alone. It had Thought to keep it company.

The duo went about their life joined at the hip for many years. When Emily felt down, Thought was right there. When Emily was feeling happy Thought was right there too. Every time perfectly matched to the way she was feeling. She had a perfect balance, she had feelings AND she had Thought.

Over time Emily came to believe her thoughts even more and her thoughts began to dominate more and more. She stopped doing things for herself and instead relied on her good old friend who had been with her all of her life.

She began to notice that sometimes Thought told her to do things that she didn't really agree with or didn't want to do but she trusted Thought so much that she went with it anyway. After all Thought always knew best. As more time passed, Emily found herself in situations that she had never imagined that she would get into. Her life was not remotely the way she had intended it to be; sometimes she wondered how that had happened? She was overweight, in a job she didn't love and in a relationship that left her unfulfilled. She reacted quickly and rashly to situations and was often doing things before she even realised it. Things that she knew she didn't really want to do.

Emily began to feel more and more frustrated and started to take her frustration out on Thought. She wished Thought would just shut up and leave her alone, sometimes she just couldn't get Thought out of her head and so she just gave into what Thought wanted (after all, that was the only way to make it stop). She would eat when Thought told her – she would drink too much because that drowned out Thought; but really she believed that Thought did know best it was just that she didn't like what she heard sometimes. Part of her knew it was wrong but she just couldn't help herself.

Then one day something happened. Emily read a book. It was as if the author was speaking just to her – he must be, he even knew her friend 'Thought'! At first Emily wasn't sure about the book, the author wasn't being very nice about her friend. 'Thought's helped me all my life,' she thought, 'Thought is my friend'. But Emily was still curious to explore, as she had always been. She had long suspected that there must be a secret, a way that other people, skinny, happy people knew so she read on … As Emily read she began to think in a different way. Could it be that, instead of having feelings AND thought, she had those feelings BECAUSE of Thought? Wow, has Thought really been running my life all this time? Have I been making decisions without noticing, just because of Thought?

What happened to *me*? What happen to what I want? What happened to my dreams? At first she dismissed it but then the more she thought the more she became angry. 'Thought has ruined my life.' 'It's all Thought's fault'. She felt betrayed and hurt and banished Thought from her life forever!

After all, how she could ever trust Thought again? How could she ever trust anything again? How would she make a decision if she didn't have Thought to tell her how to feel and what to do? She began to feel a little lost, a little vulnerable and confused. She sat back, took a deep breath and closed her eyes 'What will I do now?' she thought. And, in that moment, she realised that thought was still there, but it was different, – she had been the one 'doing' the thinking. Wow, that was cool! It sounded just like her old 'friend' but it was different. This time she had chosen the thought. Wow, I can choose my thoughts, can I really?

As she relaxed she noticed in the darkness that Thought was still there and chirping away in exactly the same way it had always been. The pictures were there, the words were there and that little voice within was still there too, but now she was not connected to Thought in the same way.

There was a kind of distance between them. They were no longer hand in glove, no longer joined at the hip. Thought was still there, spouting its wisdom but Emily could see Thought for what it was, 'it's just a thought' and she could pay attention or not, but that was her free choice, she was free! Thought happens independently of you, just like even though you are not watching TV right now, the shows are still on but you're not tuned into them.

You could engage by tuning in and casually flicking through your thoughts or you could choose to pay attention to the one in particular that makes you feel good.

That is the one which will move you and affect you. Through the attention that you give that thought, you will feel the feelings it brings. Feelings BECAUSE you tune into the thought; good feelings that you can choose at any moment – all you have to do is just sit and notice that your thoughts exist outside of you, you do not control them but you can choose which ones to let affect you. Thoughts will always be there but you don't have to let them stretch your spring out of shape.

The true power is in you the thinker, not in the thoughts.

Emily, just like you, had never thought about it this way and I'll tell you that neither had I until my friend Michael Neill (we spoke about him earlier, and you'll find more of his work on the web site) pointed it out to me. I remember arriving in LA and, on the drive to his house, Michael started to explain the ideology behind this. Perhaps it was jet lag, perhaps I'm just not very bright but I have to confess that at first I didn't get it. I didn't even realise that I had thoughts like that. Obviously I had thoughts but when I reacted to things it all happened SO quickly that I was not 'aware' of my thoughts. That said, once it was pointed out to me, I spent many a sleepless night on the web and reading books on the principles of The Psychology of Mind (jet lag again) or as it's sometimes called, 'health realisation'. I like this idea, as it implies that health is there, all you have to do is realise it now.

You know the exercise around this already, 'just sitting,' but I don't want you to get too hung up on the technique. Just acknowledging that your spring wants to return to where it should be is enough for you to start to notice some phenomenal changes in your life. As Michael might put it, 'Letting go … for it!'

Letting go not only breaks the link between you and your thoughts, it creates some space in which change is possible. I'm going to make a big statement here and say that most people try to hold on too tightly to what they have or the way they are, even when they want to be different. If you hold things too fixed and rigid then, no matter how much you'd like them to change, you will not allow the scope for change to happen. In order for change to be possible, you need to stop holding on so tight.

As human beings, we tend to be very good at being 'right' and holding ourselves in our comfort zones and fixed beliefs. Often, we would rather die than be wrong or embarrassed. I actually know people who have died because they were too stubborn or embarrassed to seek medical help. I have treated people who have lost limbs because they were too stuck in their ways to stop smoking or people who have had every opportunity to make a real difference in their lives but just wouldn't allow it to happen.

You need to be flexible and make some space for the things that you want to come into your life. Let me put it this way, if you hold on too tight there is no way that you can move. Think about it this way ... Whatever you can conceive just now is bound by the limitations of your current perceptions, historical experiences and beliefs. At best it can be a limited and distorted view of what's possible.

I'd like you to imagine that there are 3 people; one is a self made multi-millionaire who has gained wealth through their own endeavours and doesn't want for anything. The other is poor, has only known struggle, hardship and suffering all of their life. And then there is you. As you sit in your life just now, I would like you to take yourself into the body and mind of the multi-millionaire and notice how he or she would think about your current situation, the opportunities you may have and the beliefs they might hold.

Then float into the body of the poor, struggling soul and notice how that mindset affects your perspective on things and the resulting beliefs, then float back into the millionaire and then when you are ready come back into you. I want you to notice that there is more than one way to think about the same thing and that difference in perspective and the difference in the place you hold your beliefs, affects not only your attitude and actions but the things that you will attract into your life. Loosening your grip on being right gives a new perspective and clear space, where change is not only possible but inevitable.

It is this space that you can fill with all of the things you want to attract into your life but first that environment must be right, (the climate must exist in which your dreams can flourish).

The garden path of least resistance

I've recently moved into a new house and to say that the garden was a mess would be an unbelievable understatement! It took 2 guys with petrol strimmers 4 days to cut the grass and I think I owe the local council a big thank you for the 190 bags of grass clippings and weeds they took away. So, with the place cleared out and the grass cut back, I had to decide what I wanted the garden to look like, what did I want to plant?

I know nothing about gardening, nothing at all, but I do know that it only makes sense to plant things that will grow here in the cold climate of the west of Scotland. There are some things that will naturally grow here, things that will actually thrive in these conditions, but also things that, if left to their own resources, wouldn't last a night.

That's not to say that I can't have those plants in my garden but I would have to create the climate in which they can survive and then really nurture them. I could also decide what I want my garden to do for me. What will give me pleasure? Sure, I might get pleasure from picking my own oranges but I can assure you that, in this climate, that would take some nurturing, not to mention the huge expense of a heated, wind proof glasshouse. However, I could get the same pleasure from looking out on a nature garden that attracts all kinds of wildlife and birds – just as much fun, far less work and much easier to maintain. Mainly because I won't have to bring birds and wildlife into my garden, they will naturally find their way here if I create the correct environment for them.

That's the same with life and the law of attraction – if you create the right environment, good things will naturally find their way into your life without all the constant effort of growing oranges!

I '*could*' create the climate where anything will grow. Some things would be more natural than others but anything will grow if the conditions are right and you nurture it with your thoughts, love and attention.

HEALTHY

The field of quantum physics teaches us that all things are energy. Nothing really has solid form so, at some level, things and thoughts are the same thing. Let me explain. All matter (even you and I) is made up of atoms and atoms at the most basic level are really wave lengths of energy. So, at its most basic scientific level matter is really just energy flowing and vibrating at a certain frequency. Different frequency = different matter. Scientists have proven that thought can be measured, thought has and is energy and thought has a wavelength. So, if both matter and thought at their most basic level take the form of wavelengths of energy, then surely it is possible to influence matter with thought?

Bet you didn't think you'd be studying quantum physics to shed a few pounds? You don't have to but it helps to understand at this level that how we think affects the things around us. So here's the fun part ... We know that we are springs who get pulled out of shape by our thoughts and that once we detach from reacting to our thoughts, we go back to our natural healthy happy state. How would it be if you could attract things into your life just by using the power of thought in a new way? That would be way cool right? And you can!

The secret is to let yourself be the natural you and use your thoughts to bring things that you want into your life. This is not the same as just wishing. The law of attraction is always happening. What you focus on, you tend to get more of.

11 | Bonus DIFY

If you're sceptical and I know I was when I was first introduced to this idea, set yourself a small goal and enjoy making that happen first. How about making it nothing to do with weight loss for now and setting out to attract an extra £50 into your life? Not from somewhere that you know. Just from somewhere. I don't want you to know where that extra money is going to come from now, just create the climate to attract it, set the intention and allow whatever is going to happen to happen. You'll be amazed how quickly it can show up when you least expect it.

If £50 isn't a good goal for you, just set your intention on something else that works for you and go with that. Make a note in your journal and date it. It'll be fun to cross it off very soon.

Energy flows where attention goes. All things are energy and that energy will be drawn to where you put your attention. Focus on what you want, NOT what you don't want. Focusing on being slim is very different from not being fat or even losing weight. You see, the brain cannot process a negative, so if I ask you not to picture yourself wearing a blue hat, the only way you can do that is to picture yourself in the blue hat and then take the hat away. You can try that now (picture yourself without a blue hat on). Whatever you focus on you tend to get more of, so please focus on what you want.

HEALTHY

The mistake that most people make is that they don't have the right environment to start with. Most people can grasp the concept of using their thoughts to attract things; most people have had an experience of thinking of something and it showing up in their life. Have you ever thought of someone and they've called you out of the blue? Or really set your heart on something and from nowhere it just appears? The key to sustaining this state is that first you have to create the right climate or environment for your thoughts to be able to manifest and then flourish. Just like in my garden. In order for me to attract wildlife in for my enjoyment I must create the garden our furry and feathered friends would want to hang out in.

It wouldn't matter how much I wished for squirrels and birds and badgers, if my garden was a concrete mess, they are not likely to show up and even less likely to stay. Sure, I could work really hard and go out and find all those creatures and bring them to my garden but you can be sure that as soon as they could they'd be off.

Have you ever noticed that you sometimes struggle and strive really hard to get the things that you want in your life then, just as soon as you've got them, they're gone again? If you really want more money, you might have a lucky break and have a bit of extra cash, but how long does it take for normal service to be resumed, the money gone and you being back to where you started? Not long, eh?

The problem is that you do not have an environment your dreams want to hang out in. I know it's a weird idea but I can assure you that it's true. You only have to look at the number of lottery winners and other overnight windfall successes who have lost it all and returned to almost exactly the same lifestyle they had before very very quickly. In fact, only this morning I read in the newspaper of a guy who won over £10,000,000 on the lottery but is now £2,000,000 in debt and has been made bankrupt. While this is obviously a tough time for him and his family you have to think that the money didn't just disappear by itself. His losses are a result of his choices which are a direct result of the quality of his thinking and the decisions he made.

If the environment is not right, your dreams are not likely to want to hang out with you.

Some of you might be thinking that the story of my garden is just a metaphor. It is but it's also a very true example of both the principles you're learning about here. You see, I'm lucky enough to live in a wonderful house overlooking a valley and when I looked out of the window this morning, 2 squirrels were playing on the decking in my garden and a buzzard was circling majestically overhead soaring on the air currents (I don't think it spotted the squirrels ... Wonder where the second one is, hmmm?)

All very nice for a Sunday morning but the even cooler part is that I was a visitor to the house I now live in many years ago, although then I parked outside. I didn't dare to park in the driveway, it seemed way too impressive for the little car I had at the time. I thought – 'One day!' I remember it so well but the weird thing I remember noticing at the time was that I had a feeling, almost like an energetic connection to the house. Sure, I wished that one day it would be mine but I also felt it too.

I remember telling a few people about how fab the house was but I never really gave it a second thought. Then, on Christmas Day last year I decided to look for a new pad, somewhere in the countryside, away from the hustle of the city and perhaps closer to my hometown. I went on the web and did a quick search; the first house that came up was the one I am sitting in right now.

First on the list, at a price I could afford and the rest is history. Cool, eh? Now a lot of things have happened since then, my practice has become much more successful I have become more skilled and I definitely earn more money, but even so, what are the chances?

There is no amount of planning, plotting or scheming that could be done to make this happen the way it did. It's just not possible and yet these things happen every day to thousands of people, just like you and I. You can dismiss them as coincidences if you like but, when you can actually control and predict when they happen, it's a little more than a coincidence.

You see it's a bit like this. Most success and happiness books that I've read focus on 'doing', do more of this and less of that. And, if you're Scottish, then your ancestors' Calvinist programming will be ringing in your ears. Work hard, don't have too much fun. Life is hard and if you are lucky, you may be rewarded one day but probably not and then you die! I'm hoping you're not in this bracket but I can assure you that I was for many years.

For most of my adult life, the equation was very simple in my head. Hard Work + Hope = Success. I didn't know what success looked like but I wanted it and was prepared to work my butt off to get it. I had no idea where I was going but I was in a hurry to get there!

I worked and I worked and I worked and, if what I was working at didn't work out, I would try something else and work and work and work at that! Boy, was it tiring!

I know some of you will be wondering what this has to do with weight loss, well it's simple. Being overweight is as much an emotional state as it is a physical state. In order to change your waistline for good we need to focus on the space between your ears. That way, you will keep the weight off for good. I don't want you to be the one scooping the top prize through graft and struggle just to put all the weight back on again. That's not the deal, you've got to allow it to be as easy as you can. This is about making changes for good.

So back to my little story. I remember telling someone (bragging actually) that I had worked 28 days straight without a break. I was exhausted but I was proud of my effort and wore it like a badge of honour, hoping I would be rewarded one day. How wrong was I? As I look back on that time now, I can't even remember what it was that I was trying to achieve, and I can assure you that the rewards are not sitting in my bank account to remind me. I was working hard but stupidly. Success can be effortless if you allow it to be. That doesn't mean you can just sit back and expect good things to flow towards you but you can let go of the emotional pain and struggle.

By controlling what we can on the inside, we can influence things on the outside.

The secret you see is not in the 'doing' but in creating a space of 'being' in which you can attract and keep what you want. If that sounds a little weird, let me explain.

Remember my garden? The one with the lone squirrel and lots of birds? Well, my garden doesn't 'do' anything to attract the wildlife, just' 'being' there is enough. The garden doesn't work hard to get what I want in it. I put all the effort in long ago creating it and now it just 'is' and what I want is attracted to it. In this example, you can see that it's really simple. If I want wildlife in my garden, I create the garden to attract and maintain wildlife.

The same is true with your life. If you want to attract good things into your life (and get to enjoy them for some time) you have to create an environment where this is not just possible but inevitable (if you think inevitable is too strong, you try and keep blackbirds away from your raspberries).

It feels a little odd at first when the things you want start to show up in your life. You'll be forgiven for thinking 'Oh, that was lucky' or 'What a cool coincidence' but it's not luck and not a coincidence, it's the way it can be.

Think about it this way, you'd love to have all your friends in the same place at the same time to really enjoy spending time together. Now if your friends are anything like mine, it can be a bit like herding cats.

So, you could either;

- Set about doing it the hard way and use all your powers of persuasion to force them to cancel their other plans and come along.
Or
- you could do it the easy way. You see the secret to herding cats is that it's easy if you have a large enough mouse.

Create a wonderful environment and then invite people to join you in it.

It's exactly the same with all the things you want to attract into your life. Create the right environment. That is, set the quality of your thinking and then please remember to invite things to show up. Then, listen out for your inner wisdom and follow it wherever it may lead.

You can do this first by stopping trying so hard, stop focusing on the struggle and just allow yourself to 'be' happy. Allow yourself to re-connect with the wisdom that is within you.

I know that you already know when you are going against your inner knowing, you know when something just doesn't feel quite right but the trick is to stop, notice and do something about it … Follow your heart and your intuition. It knows far more than you think.

Ok, so from now on I'm going to be your coach. I'm going to approach this in exactly that same way as if you were sitting in my office with me. (Ok, you might get a cup of tea if you were with me but make your own and you'll feel at home.)

Let me ask you a few questions ... Just note your answers in your head or your journal.

What do you really want?
How will you know when you have that?
What would you wish for even if you didn't think you could get it?
What is the biggest thing that is holding you back?
What is the simplest choice you can make that will release you to move towards your dreams?
Why are you ready to move forward now?
Why is this time different?
What have you have learned so far that you think will make the biggest difference in our life?
How much do you love me? ... Just testing to see if you're still awake ... Tee Hee! ☺

All of this is to serve one purpose. To let you live life on your terms for a change. How much would you love to be slim, fit and healthy? You can and you know how already. I hope that you have been jotting things down in your journal and really getting stuck into making a difference in your life. It's amazing just how quickly things can change when you let them.

I am constantly amazed at what we can achieve in a single year. When I look back over the last year it feels like no time at all and yet looking forward to the next

12 months feels like an eternity. Just stop and have a think about this time last year. What were you doing? Where were you on this day last year? If you keep a diary, look back and see. If not, just have a good guess. Doesn't it feel like 5 minutes ago. Now, how about this time next year? What will you be doing? What will you look like? How will your life be different? What are you looking forward to most? When in that year will you know you have achieved what you set out to achieve? How good does that feel?

We have reached the end of Slim Fit and Healthy, please just take a few moments to reflect on your journal and notice how far you have come already and give yourself a moment to feel good about that. Perhaps you'd like to pick out some of your favourite DIFY sections and play with them again? Or maybe you'd prefer to just reflect on what you have learned and how it can feel very different.

12 | Bonus DIFY – Pay a compliment

Some people are so stingy with them you would think they cost the earth! Pay compliments to people and get used to accepting them in return. This will help you to shift your thinking from 'woe is me and everyone else is ok' to a more loving, giving and receiving place where things can flow into 'your' life and you can enjoy them when they do.

HEALTHY

Here's the exercise. I want you to find a reason to talk to and pay a sincere compliment to 3 strangers today. It doesn't have to be cheesy or gushy, just notice when you notice something that you appreciate and instead of keeping it to yourself or even feeling jealous or envious, pay that person a nice sincere compliment.

You'll be amazed at the effect it has on … You! And for them, of course, but that's just a bonus!

When you've done that you'll be ready to get active. This is where we take all you have done so far and really go for it … Let's make some dreams come true!

Active

Argh!! We've got to the active bit ... This *must* be the part where the lycra comes out again!!??

Erm, well, sorry to disappoint you but it's not. Or at least not because I say so – you're more than welcome to pull on your leotard and keep reading if you want, it'll be our little secret.

This is the fun part, this is the part of the book where you get to 'Ooh and ahh!' a lot.

We're going to play a little game. Let's call our game 'the game of my life', after all what's the point of life if it's not fun? I want you to view the next section as being about having fun!! Having fun AND making your dreams come true at the same time. This is how it works.

If you enjoy something you will tend to do more of it. If you do more, you tend to get better at it and, if you are getting better and better at it, you will tend to enjoy it more and do even more of it ... Makes sense right?

So, where do you start in that process? Well, no matter what it is you're doing, I will always suggest you start with 'enjoying it'. It doesn't matter what it is, I want you to find ways to get more enjoyment out of what you are doing.

As you sit reading this, what could you do to enjoy it more? Could you make yourself a little more comfortable in your chair? Could you think some happy thoughts? Or, could you keep in mind why you are doing this and just how fabulous you are going to feel when you are slim, fit, healthy and enjoying being active in your life?

ACTIVE

Maybe you can really go for it and do all 3 now, or, just as soon as you like.

I have included this section as, to my mind, this is the whole point of the work you have done so far. Slim, Fit, Healthy, for what? Well, this is the 'For what' section. What is it that the slimmer, fitter, healthier **you** would like to take action to 'be' or 'do' or 'have' for that matter now?

If you like, this is the goal setting section. This is the part where you get to make your dreams come true. Sorry, you'll not find the winning lottery numbers here but you might hit the jackpot just the same.

It doesn't matter if you are rich or poor, young or old or anywhere in between. You can enjoy the satisfaction of setting goals and achieving them. Now before we start, let me give you my take on goal setting – it's a little different from most.

You may well have heard elsewhere that goals must be SMART, that is to say they must be Specific, Measurable, Achievable, Realistic and with a Time frame. That sounds more like a business plan to me … your goals should be FUN!

Goals should be the things that make you come alive; goals and dreams should be the things that make you feel warm and fuzzy when you think about them. I was working with an internationally renowned coach recently. We were in the Middle East discussing how he was putting together a huge coaching project that will likely change the face of business in one of the Gulf States.

When I asked him how he was going about it, he said 'I'm finding where the energy is and going with that'. In other words, he was building a multi million pound business which will affect the economy of an entire country on the basis of where people's passions and energies lay. (On what makes the people involved come alive.) Wow, that was kind of cool …

It reminded me of a quote by Howard Thurman **'Don't ask yourself what the world needs. Ask yourself what makes you come alive, and go do that, because what the world needs is people who have come alive'.**

So, how do you know what you really want to do? Easy, it's the thing that gives you that fuzzy glow of excitement that feels like it effortlessly drives you forward.

Goals are the things that make you fall more deeply in love with your life. And the pursuit of goals can be effortless, or at least it can feel that way. That's a true goal. Anything else is just a plan. Does that make sense? Where will your passion take you?

In the earlier section, we have already said you don't have to know specifically how to get what you want, you don't have to plan and methodically plot your progress, you just need to create the climate that attracts what you want and allow it to happen. Remember, I didn't have a clue how to go about getting the house of my dreams, yet I'm sitting in it now writing this for you.

I have coined the phrase 'effortless effort' to illustrate what I mean here. It's a cool way of checking if what you are working towards is really a wow goal or just something that might be good for now.

Effortless effort – The state where nothing is too much trouble.

The idea of effortless effort first came to me years ago when I was working with a client. My client was a very big name in the personal development world and I was over the moon to be working with him. I was his Personal Fitness Trainer. I was there to motivate and guide someone to whom thousands of people looked up and respected. How cool is that?

The only small problem was that my client was obviously very busy and the only time he could see me was first thing in the morning, 6.30am, ok so far … at his house … which was a good 90 minute drive from mine, fine … and it was winter … and I had a Mini! And, he wasn't paying me..!

I know many Personal Trainers who would have laughed in my face at the thought of taking that deal, but I didn't just take it, I relished it! Up at 4.30 am twice a week to drive to his house and put him through his paces … Fantastic! I loved it! Why? Because in doing so, I was making one of my dreams come true. I was working with one of the best in the world and I loved it. I certainly wasn't doing it for the financial gain. Once I had paid for my petrol, it was actually costing me money but it was worth every penny.

Effortless effort has been demonstrated to me many, many times by friends, family and clients over the years.

Have you ever been in love with someone who lives far away? The long journey to see them, even if it is just for a short while feels effortless. Have you followed your team home and away, travelling the length and breadth of the country and relishing it? Or, when you are doing something that you really love the time flies by and it doesn't feel like work? How cool would it be to have that every day?

Someone once told me to 'find something you're good at and make a living out of it' I found that I was really good at talking people to sleep … !

Ok, so let's find out where your effortless effort sits.

What is it that when you think about doing it, the thought just makes you light up? What is it that brings a real smile to your face and that the thought of it just feels so good now?

I'd like you to quickly make a list of things you'd love to 'be,' 'do' or 'have', whether you think you can have them or not … Nothing logical here, nothing that would be a logical step from where you are now. This is the big stuff. This is where you get to really dream. No one will see your dreams and, if you've kept what you're doing just between us for now, then no one will ask you about them either. This is where you can just kick back and relax and dare to dream again.

ACTIVE

What do you want to be when you grow up?

People grow old but seldom truly grow up, not really in themselves. You probably act differently because of the way society expects you to be, but I'm guessing that if you're like me you still feel like a teenager at heart. Sometimes we get a glimpse of that when we hear a song that takes us back to those carefree days. They didn't feel like it at the time but when you look back now you will realise that you very rarely see things for what they are when you are in them. And that is just as true of you today. No matter how stuck you might feel, you only have to think of how far you have come to know that you are always on a journey. Only now, you get to set the direction.

People think that I spend my time putting people into trance. I actually spend most of my time waking people up from the trance they have been in for most of their lives. People go through life on auto pilot – the problem being that they are not the ones programming it. Now you can wake up from your state and set about shaping the future of you and for you, in a very personal way.

I was recently doing a radio interview to coincide with the launch of the film *The Bucket List*. If you've not seen the movie, it's about 2 guys from very different backgrounds who find themselves thrown together in the same hospital ward, both with incurable cancer. Morgan Freeman's character has no money but he still has unfulfilled dreams so he creates his 'bucket list', things he wants to do before he … well, kicks the bucket. Jack

THE SLIM GIRL'S BOOK OF SECRETS

Nicholson's character has loads of money but nothing to live for, so the pair set off on a quest to tick off all the items on the list. This got me thinking, what would be on my list?

'Why wait till you're dying to start living your life?'

As I thought a bit more about it, I realised that all of the things I would put on my list fell neatly into three categories.

The person I'd like to BE
What I'd like to DO
What I'd like to HAVE

So, what are the things that you want to BE, DO or HAVE whether you think you can have it or not ...

BE

_____

_____

_____

DO

_____

_____

_____

HAVE

_____

_____

_____

ACTIVE

Please don't let me limit you, take more space if you need it ...

Now, have a look at your goals and ask yourself 'What would I be prepared to do to get this? Just jot it down beside the goal.

Now, have a look at those answers again and notice if the thing you were prepared to do was 'giving up or doing without' something else?

You'll often hear people saying things like, "I'd give my eye teeth to have" ... or "I'd give my left arm to be able to play like her". (I'm guessing that wouldn't really help)

Now what I want you to do is to go back through your answers and correct them to 'What would you be prepared to do to get it?'

BE   Positively prepared to do about it

_____

_____

DO

_____

_____

_____

HAVE

_____

_____

_____

Cool – Now I'll assume that all of the above are legal and that I'm not encouraging you to get into trouble in any way.

Your goals in your life

Ok, so we've got some well formed, specific goals? Now it's time to build your life around them.

We're all different and we will all have very different goals and aspirations but I have given you a bit of a head start by listing some of the main areas of life that my clients normally come to me with issues in. It may be that you are wanting to focus on one of these or you may need a little nudge with them all to differing degrees. I would suggest, however, that for now, you pick the 3 parts that feel right to you. Some suggestions are …

Health, Weight, Relationships, Money, Career, Something bigger than me. But you can fill in the ones that feel most relevant to you right now. I say parts because they are just that, parts of a whole and although an area in need of attention can feel all consuming, it is just part of the greater whole that is you. Let me give you an example.

Give yourself a score for each from 1–10 as to where you are relative to where you would love to be.

First just note down what 0 would mean to you.

ACTIVE

E.g. **The <u>relationships</u> part of my life**

```
0                                                    10
```

0 = The pits

> Alone, un-
> loved and
> lonely

You might be wondering why I want you to put the worst possible score on your scale, well, for 2 reasons really.

1. To give a sense of perspective
2. It is often useful before you start setting new goals to just realise where you are now and how far you are along the scale already. Give yourself a pat on the back and acknowledge that you are wonderful, talented and special and that you, and you alone, shape your life and dreams.

Take a breather – take a few moments to just be grateful for what you have and for who you are and for all you have achieved so far.

Before we move on, let's have a good look at where you're at now. Very soon it will be time to move on to the next phase of your life and really start living up to your full potential but for now just take a few moments to close your eyes and say thank you to whoever or whatever is listening in your world for all that you have and all that is good and all that you are enriched by ... go ahead, enjoy taking time to pause and say thanks. Remember to thank yourself because it's you who has done this and you can still do so much more too.

Where you are now?
What is interesting in this part is the way you describe where you are now ... Just pick a part of your life and write what comes to mind and then notice what that says about you and your dreams ... Re-read this again and notice what you notice about the way you describe where you are currently. What might be stopping you from going further?

E.g. **The relationships part of my life**

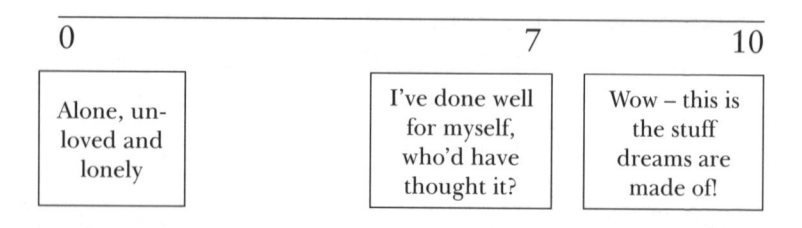

0	7	10
Alone, un-loved and lonely	I've done well for myself, who'd have thought it?	Wow – this is the stuff dreams are made of!

I'd like you to take a few minutes and just fill in the blanks for each of these headings. For the 'Wow, this is the stuff dreams are made of', don't just write what you think you can have, write down what would make you feel like a child on Christmas morning who's just found out that Santa has broken down outside their house. (Probably should have said Santa's sleigh has broken

ACTIVE

down, the idea of Santa having a breakdown outside your house is probably not so cool, but you know what I mean). Really go for it! What's the point of dreaming if you're not going to really go for it?

The <u>relationships</u> part of my life

0	7	10
Alone, un-loved and lonely	I've done well, who'd have thought it?	Loving, high intimacy, low maintenance relationship.

Now do the same for each of your 3 'parts':

1 The _____ part of my life

0   10

2 The _____ part of my life

0   10

3 The _____ part of my life

0   10

There is a weird phenomenon that works to bring into your life what you focus on, we chatted about it earlier. Now the cool thing about this is that, even if you don't get your Wow, 10 out of 10, you might get a good 9, which would only have been a 4 or a 5 if you'd been dreaming of mediocre.

There is something about stretching the thermostat of our expectation which helps us to put a new perspective on things. I remember working with a client who wanted to make more money. He was already fully booked and was charging a daily fee of about £100 but he couldn't physically do any more hours so I suggested that he put his fees up. 'I can't' he said. 'Why not?' 'Because I'm not comfortable with asking for more and besides I don't think anyone will pay more'. I quickly asked him if he knew of anyone in his field who charged more than he did and, of course, the answer was yes. So, the only thing stopping him from having more was him. Or, to be more accurate, his limiting belief about what he was worth.

Know your own worth (have a play with this for anything you like, here we're going to play for money as my client did)

Have a think about how much you think you are worth. How much are you worth in terms of your annual salary? That's not how much you currently get paid but how much do you feel you are worth. Write the number down here £ _____ per annum

This is what I did with my client …

Ok, so you want to make more money. So, just close your eyes and try on the idea of asking a client for £1,000 per day, that's ten times what you charge now'. He thought for a moment then said 'No way, I can't see myself doing that, it feels like way too much'. 'Ok, try £800 per day'. Again, 'Too much'. We did this all the way down to £250 where he said 'Hmmm, that feels better, I can see myself doing that fairly comfortably'.

His homework, you'll not be surprised to learn, was to quote £250 per day the next time someone asked him his fees. Do you know that 2 days later he called me to say he received a call from a new client and had just booked 2 days of work at his new fee. And the client didn't even flinch at the price.

Why am I telling you this story? Well for 2 reasons really.

1. Before you do anything you have to be congruent, comfortable and believe in what you are doing and what you are worth. Otherwise it will show through and neither you, nor the person you are asking for the money, will feel comfortable.
2. By cranking my client's financial thermostat all the way up, we had changed the scale on which his brain was functioning. £250 on a scale of £100 to £1,000 is a lot less than £250 on a scale of £100 to £500. What we had actually done was to increase his fee by 250%, yet it felt more comfortable because we had first gone to a number much, much bigger and worked our way back. The same is true in your life with anything you

want. He was delighted with his new fee and went on to fill his order book and make a lot more money for the same or even less effort. The same can be true for you. If you set your sights high and fall halfway short, you're still a lot better off than if you set your sights low.

3. Play with this for yourself and then write your new self worth here _____ Remember it can be in terms of money, love, career or anything else you care to measure.

You wouldn't believe what's holding you back.
Imagine you are going for a new job and the salary for the new job is £10,000 more than you currently earn. I'll let you do the maths here.

Current salary/annual income £ _____ (Figure A)
New job is £10,000 more so £ _____ (Figure B)
How do you feel about your £10,000 pay rise? _____

As you sit in the office before your interview, the boss's PA hands you your new job description and you notice that the job doesn't pay £10,000 more, it pays 10 times more. (Add a zero to Figure A) How do you feel about it now as you sit there waiting for the interview? I'll bet that if you weren't nervous already, you certainly are now.

I have worked with clients who would simply have got up and left at that point because it was too big for them (maybe that would have been you?) More money

ACTIVE

than they could ever dream of and yet they would walk away, or think 'what's the catch'? You see, often it's not the lack of money, love, confidence, health or energy that is holding you back – it's your attitude to it. This isn't just true with money, it's true in all areas of our lives. More often than not, the thing holding you back is in fact not real – it's the idea you hold about it.

13 | DIFY – Turn your worth all the way up

We all have an idea of ourselves, who we are, what we stand for and, strangely, a concept of what we are worth. Although I know when you write it like that it doesn't sit quite right. You know the kind of thing, 'He's out of my league' or 'Don't get above your station' or 'That's not for the likes of me' or any of the other well worn phrases we use to put and keep ourselves down.

Strangely, we also use phrases like 'I'm not worthy' or we are said to 'undervalue' ourselves. The idea of self worth comes from fear, fear of failure usually but often a fear of success.

How would it be if you really did feel priceless or rich in every way or maybe settled or content or satisfied would be the way you would like to describe yourself. These are all common ways of doing it and I'm not saying they are wrong but I would love for you to try doing it a different way. How about if you were already like that?

Already, exactly as you'd love to be, already there. I'd love you to consider that the journey to get there is not forward but back. It's not so much about re-programming as re-setting. Pressing the re-set button and allowing you to be the authentic you. Who is the authentic you? Where is the authentic you? What does the authentic you love to do? What skills and capabilities does the authentic you have? What values does that the authentic you hold most dear?

It's ok to be you! I think you'll like the authentic you a whole lot better. I'd like you to just sit for a minute or two and ask yourself the following questions.

Where is the authentic me? _____
What does the authentic me do? _____
What skills does the authentic me have? _____
What beliefs and values does the authentic me hold? _____

What is beyond the authentic me? _____
What is it that flows through me, not from me, that carries the authentic me? _____

As you do this, you will notice you can enjoy a wonderful feeling of peace and calm and that, well, it's ok to be you. You are ok and the world is a better place because of you.

I'd first of all like you to work through different parts of your life or just the ones you worked with earlier and note in your journal which areas you are not being 'authentic' in or not living your values.

Take each in turn and just note, what is it about that area that's not authentic? How do you know that?

Now here you know better than me. For each of your answers, What is the simplest thing you know to do to bring this back into living in a place of authenticity? You know best, What is the best thing you can do to help yourself in each of these areas right now?

Work through each and write down your answers. Now, ask yourself a very simple question.

What stops me? _____

Ok, by working through that stuff and bringing yourself back to neutral you now have a fabulous place to start designing a wonderful and fulfilling life.

So, what I'd like you to do now is to work through your life areas and note what 'Wow, this is the stuff dreams are made of' means to you. Do not limit yourself. I have seen pub singers top the charts, bankrupts become millionaires and all kinds of people live a life they have only dreamed of … This is your turn.

BUT … this is not about working hard, this is about having fun! This is not about struggle and grafting to get what you want, this is about letting go and just going for it. It really can be that easy if you let it.

Remember, it doesn't take a lot of effort to get your spring back to its original shape but you do have to be prepared to let go and allow yourself to just be.

Who do you want to be?

I'd like you to PLAY with the next section. Just play with it and see what happens. Play doesn't mean "don't do it," it genuinely means play with it. Do you remember going out to play when you were little? My friends and I took playtime seriously ...

I think I used to pretend I was Pelé when we were playing football or Boris Becker when we were playing tennis. I'm not sure if kids still do that now but 'who' you were was just as fiercely contested as the game itself. You see, although I didn't realise it at the time I got satisfaction, confidence and pleasure out of the association with 'who' I 'was'. If I 'was' Pelé, I would run a bit faster or play with more flair (probably just in my head) but it felt better. I know that a few years ago the daughter of a friend was playing with some friends at 'being' the Spice Girls. The roles were hotly contested, whoever got to be Scary was the leader and Sporty would run around while Posh would pout a lot and hang out where the boys played football. Just kidding Victoria!

You see it doesn't matter who you are but the idea you hold of yourself does. It wasn't that I took on any of the strength or skill of Pelé but I did feel like I had a little bit of him in me. So, actually it wasn't that I was Pelé, but more that my idea of Pelé was in me.

When you go out to play with this section who are you going to be?

Here's the deal – you will get the chance to 'be' your heroes in every part of your life. Sounds fun? Ok, let's find out ...

Let's split the next bit into the same sections of your life as before ... Who are you going to be? I know you're

ACTIVE

thinking you're too old for this but again just run with me on it, it'll be fun.

When we let go of our limiting belief and the idea we hold of ourselves, we can borrow a little from other people, after all, isn't that what we do logically when we learn anything? We get to share the knowledge of someone else, so why can't we do that emotionally and step into the shoes of who you are going to be? Or, who is going to 'be' in you.

Take your 3 areas from page 171 and just write them in the boxes again.

Part 1 e.g.	Part 2	Part 3
The relationship part		
_____	_____	_____
The Beckhams		
....	....	....
Goldie Hawn & Kurt Russell		
....	....	....
My friends Andy & Susan		
....	....	....
Heidi Klum & Seal and of course Brad & Angelina		
....	....	....
....	....	....

Now – for each one I'd like you make a list of all the people you know (or know of) who are possible candidates. People who you'd like to play you in this area. This is not about you becoming them, this is about them helping you from the inside.

I want you to try the idea of Audrey Hepburn's sense of style inside you as a 'get ready for a night out' or the idea of Madonna inside you when you need to be confident or Sir Richard Branson helping you from the inside in business. These people will be more or less themselves but in your life. I know this might be bit of a bonkers idea but in my experience it works really well.

It's not that you are going to become them. In my experience that doesn't work terribly well. It's difficult to associate with someone who is incredibly good at something and so far removed from your life. But borrowing some of the essence of what makes them successful works brilliantly. How would it be if instead of you stepping into Audrey Hepburn, you took the essence of her into you. After all, isn't this what happened when I was playing at 'being' Pelé at football or you are being 'Madonna' on the Karaoke or being anyone else for that matter? You are trying to emulate them. To make like them but within your life. It's a lot easier to change from the inside out than the outside in.

So I'd like you to first make a list of all the candidates for the part of 'you'. If one of the areas of your life you'd like to work on is confidence you might like to have … Madonna or Beyoncé or Sienna Miller or Oprah Winfrey on your list. Or, if the area you are working on is

ACTIVE

Finances, you might like to have Donald Trump or Duncan Bannatyne or Sir Richard Branson on your casting list. And for now that's what it is, it's a casting list. A list of possible talent. Get the idea?

Now it doesn't have to be famous people, just people whose qualities you would like to have. Or, if it helps you, just imagine that the playground game is finance or confidence or love – who do you want to 'be'?

Ok, so go ahead and make your list of who you might be going to be … do it for each of the 3 areas and, when you're done, we'll be ready to move on.

Beside each of the candidates, jot down a note of what it is about that person that has earned them their place on your list. Why are they on your short list? Be specific here, what is it about Madonna that make you want to 'be' her and feel good about that. Or what is it that makes you want to 'be' Sir Richard Branson. Why would you feel proud if you 'were' Sienna Miller in the playground game of style? Make your list first then go back and add in your 'whys'

The _____ part of my life

Who_____ why _____

Who_____ why _____

Who_____ why _____

Who_____ why _____

The _____ part of my life

Who_____ why _____

Who_____ why _____

Who_____ why _____

Who_____ why _____

The _____ part of my life

Who_____ why _____

Who_____ why _____

Who_____ why _____

Who_____ why _____

Cool – so you should now have quite a list of the great and the good, and I'll guess a few great and good people you actually know too?

As you look down your list of whys, what do you notice about them? In what way are they different from you? In what way are they similar? I know that I have done this exercise with many clients and found that the qualities that they are admiring so much in others are actually qualities that they already have somewhere in themselves but maybe in a different area of their life. Acknowledge that and be thankful for it now.

If this is true of you and or even if it doesn't quite feel like it yet, I'd like you to just close your eyes and audition each person in turn. I'd like you to do it a little differently from the way you might have done this in the past.

ACTIVE

Remember you are not trying to be them. They are trying to help you.

14 | DIFY – Using all of your resources

So close your eyes and I'd like you to make a picture of that person, or just get a sense of what they are like, then focus on the quality you *specifically* admire in them and allow yourself to just try it on in you. Success is a state of mind, not an event. If, by some Act of God, they were to lose it all tomorrow, who would your money be on to get it back? Richard Branson or the lottery winner? It's all about the quality of your thinking.

Try on how it feels and how you think that person would think and how that person would look at your world. They wouldn't be critical. I'm sure they'd respect many of your qualities but there would be changes. Remember they are in you and on your side, they don't have their usual resources so they have to start from a position of your life. Try this on and notice what you notice. How does it feel to 'be' them in your life now?

Each time you find something that you really like just squeeze your finger and thumb together and take a moment to enjoy the feeling, find the best bit and really soak it up. Do this for each of the people on your list, bring them into your life and then soak up the best bit about having them inside you and on your side. Notice any insights or revelations you may have. Often we find clarity when we step out of the normal and go beyond our limiting beliefs.

You see it's not really the person but the way you think about that person, that makes you feel good. And, as you take more and more of the essence of each person, you will notice you start to feel much better in yourself and, if you feel much better in yourself now, then you can begin to go out to play as Pelé or do business as Richard Branson or have the confidence of Beyoncé.

It can be fun and you can begin to make all sorts of things happen now just because you hold the idea of who you are in a different place. A place where dreams come true and where you deserve to be happy and a place where you can attract things into your life not because I say so but just because that's the way that's right for you.

Now Anchor it …

Have you ever turned on the radio and a song has taken you back to a time and place? Or maybe you've been walking down the street and the smell of someone's perfume has instantly reminded you of someone you know? In NLP we call this Anchoring. That person is anchored to that scent or that memory is anchored to that song. You don't have to think about it consciously, the thought just comes to mind in a heart beat and there is nothing you can do about it.

This phenomenon is sometimes referred to as "triggering", in that the memory is 'triggered' by the song or smell. It's a funny thing but it happens every day to all of us and we hardly give it a second thought. We all have hundreds, if not thousands, of these anchors set up already. We didn't consciously put them there, they just kind of happened.

One of the weirdest anchors I have is that every time I head for lunch from my clinic, I have to walk by a bus stop. There are always people smoking as they wait for their bus. I'm not sure what it is about the area but there appears to be a high number of pipe smokers or maybe it's rolling tobacco, but there is something different about that smell from the smell of normal cigarettes. I guess it's sweeter. Now the weird thing is that, no matter how many times this happens, I think of my Dad. It's not that my Dad smoked a pipe or roll ups. The memory is more specific than that. It's actually a memory of standing on the terraces watching football with him when I was about 10 years old. It happens every time and while I don't like smoking, it's a lovely memory.

So, that's all very well, but what's the point of this little tale? Well, if anchors can be set that still make you feel good 20 years (ok, 24 years) after they were set, how cool would it be to set some new ones now that will make you feel good for many years to come? We actually started this in the previous section.

What we are doing here is using something which happens totally naturally but harnessing it for your benefit and giving you the chance to choose which anchors you have and when the good feelings happen. Cool eh?

Ok, so here's how it works, Our brains cannot tell the difference between imagined and reality but the more 'real' you make the imagined situation the more powerful it will feel and the stronger your anchor will be. Let me put it this way.

If this wasn't true then movies wouldn't work. We know very well that what we are watching isn't real yet we still cry at the sad bits, laugh at the funny bits and jump when we get a shock. Somehow our brain suspends the disbelief and just goes with it. At this level, it is the same as reality and the bigger the screen and the better the sound the more we become immersed in the plot line and the emotion on the screen. The bigger the better. The same movie viewed on a small portable TV or the small screen on an aeroplane would be far less powerful than the same pictures viewed at the I-Max with big sound. The purpose of the big screen and surround sound is to create feelings. Pictures and sounds = feelings. And it's the good feelings that we want here.

Big pictures + Big sounds = Big feelings

15 | DIFY – Feel good now.

So, let me help you to help yourself … What I'd like you to do first is to pick a memory that you love, one that really makes you feel good and close your eyes and bring back this memory. Now I want you to make it as real as possible in every way. Make the pictures big and bright and bold. Make sure you are seeing through your own eyes and then notice the sounds. Maybe it's sounds on

ACTIVE

the outside, like laughter or music. Or, maybe it's sounds on the inside, like thoughts, 'Ah, that's good' or 'Whoopee this is so much fun!' Now notice where the good feeling is, notice if it feels light or heavy, notice if it feels warm or cool, notice if it moves and, if so, which way? Does it move up to make it better or down? Or does it spin around now? Whatever it does for you, double it in size and then again and again until it feels great! Then ... I want you to keep that good feeling by gently pressing together any finger and the thumb on your left hand, that's right just sit and enjoy that good strong powerful feeling, then keep it by anchoring it (by pressing your finger and thumb together, told you we'd started already).

You might have to do this a few times to get a really powerful response, but once you have it, you will be able to simply press that finger and thumb together and the good feelings just start and then grow all by themselves. Just like the memory that instantly kicks in when you hear that song or my memory of my Dad. You can't stop it but you can use it to change the way you feel in any given moment ... Feel free to use your anchor any time you like.

Quick tip – Anchors don't have to be set just in your imagination. Set a good anchor now and then the next time you are out with friends, or just having a great time, squeeze that same finger and thumb together as if to say 'Ah, I'll keep this good feeling'. Try it, you'll love it!

16 | DIFY – Advanced anchoring ... Feeling even better

Now here's another cool way to use your anchor. Did you notice when you float into the person you were auditioning to 'be' you that you actually felt some of what it must feel like to 'be' them? That's totally normal and we're going to use that to our advantage. Close your eyes and pick just one of the people on your list. Make a picture of them and then bring that person into you, so that you can have the essence of them inside you now. Find the part that you like best – it might be the way they think or the way they see the world or it might be their feeling of confidence and certainty that makes you feel different.

When you have a sense of that, just take whatever is strongest for you and turn it all the way up. Make the pictures bigger and brighter and make the sounds all encompassing and the feelings stronger. Turn it all the way up – there is no limit to how strong you can make this feel. So really go for it and enjoy yourself.

I'd like you to repeat the exercise for each of the 3 focus areas you have chosen and try out your shortlist of candidates. Take the best bits from each and each time squeeze together your finger and thumb to make a powerful anchor. Now add in your favourite song by playing it in your head and turning the volume up, you can play it as loud as you like, you can't annoy the neighbours in your head.

ACTIVE

You can use this anchor anytime you like to switch on those good feelings and help you to be ... just as you want it to be.

Stylish

THE SLIM GIRL'S BOOK OF SECRETS

Ok, now I'm not going to pretend that I know anything at all about this subject (hey I'm a guy!). But I hope by now you are well on your way to enjoying a slimmer, fitter, healthier and more active life? That being the case you've probably started thinking about your new look and a new wardrobe, a trip to the shops may be in order ... Oh, you've been already?

Ok, ok I know, you don't need an excuse but hey at least now you can blame me when you get home. You have my permission to hide the packaging and the receipt and pretend you've had it for ages if you have to, but I'd love you to read this section then pop to the shops and treat yourself to something that'll help you feel great.

You don't need to break the bank either, a few, well chosen items in the right colour and style will have you feeling and looking fabulous in no time.

Let me stop for a second – this is not retail therapy! Well, not conventional retail therapy anyway. The conventional retail model is designed to make you want to buy and therefore feel happy. Spend = happy. So, here's the inside track. Just for now jot down the amount of money that you think you would have to spend in order to feel great, really great! £_____.00

It's about how you look and how you feel. Let's do a very quick exercise, come back, come back! No need for trainers ... I want you to take a minute and think of your very happiest clothed memory... I'm not being rude, oh maybe just a little but what I mean is, not your wedding day (posh frock) or the birth of your children (naked) just a memory that when you think about it makes you feel great. Got it? Good!

Quickly do a little bit of mental arithmetic and add up the rough cost of the clothes you were wearing. Have you got the amount? £_____.00 I'll bet it's a lot less than the one above, right? So it's not about the expenditure.

When I did this exercise I was astonished at just how low my number was. In my very best memory ever I have a total outfit expenditure of about £200 and that includes my rather expensive sunglasses.

'It's not about the spending – It's about the look and feel'.
As I have already said I know nothing about style. Anyone who knows me will certainly vouch for that. But, you don't have to be an expert to be able to find one and so just as I did with the fitness section, I went out and found you someone who really does know their stuff, then persuaded them to share their trade secrets with me, so that I could share them with you. Shhh ... don't tell anyone.

What you will find here is the combined wisdom of one of the top stylists in the industry and, of course, my take on the psychology behind it.

Hey, who'd have thought you'd have your very own Life Coach, Personal Trainer and Stylist. Feeling special yet?

As always the next section is tailored to fit you perfectly.

You will learn how to choose the perfect hairstyle for your face shape, how to pick the ideal clothes to flatter your figure and which colours will complement your natural skin tones. In short, all the trade secrets that the rich and famous usually like to keep to themselves. Here we'll teach you the tips and tricks of the trade to have you looking even more amazing. Who knows I might even try it myself …

To make it really easy we have broken this part down to 3 sections

Colour – Shape – Style

We're going to begin with colour. By the end of this section you will be able to go shopping with new found confidence and pick out the colours that naturally make you look great.

Colour is something we use everyday. It affects how we feel. It attracts us to food, flowers and each other. Imagine a world without colour?

Let me show you just how much colour adds to your experience of the world. Take a moment to close your eyes and bring back your favourite happy memory, make the picture big and bright and bold. Rate how good it feels on a scale from 1–10. Now, just for a second drain the colour completely out of the picture and make the picture black and white. Rate it again now … Quite a difference, eh? Ok, put the colour back in now before you imagine bland food like Cauliflower, Potatoes, Pasta, all on the same plate. Even if you knew it tasted great you probably wouldn't order it.

We all like to feel special and look good when we go out, so the more colour we can inject the better. Let me quickly qualify that, I do not want you going out looking like an explosion in a paint factory. Let's find the colour combinations that really work *for* you. The colours we choose should compliment our natural skin tone or 'undertone'

When we are wearing a colour that best suits our personal undertone, it can make you look younger, healthier and most importantly of all make you feel great.

Our skin undertone is genetic, something we are born with and cannot change. We inherit it from our parents and so we have to work with our natural colouring, not against it.

It doesn't matter how expensive an outfit is, if it's wrong, it's wrong! A quick flick through any of the many celebrity magazines will show you that even the celebs get it very wrong too.

Throughout this section you will learn how to analyse your own colour yourself, then we'll go through a few exercises you can go out and have some fun with. Hey, shopping can be even more fun! As if you needed that …

All you will need to get started is a bright, naturally lit room, a mirror by the window, a chair and the sample colours you will find in your Box of Secrets. We're going to begin here, once you've got your colour sorted it's a piece of cake from there …(pardon the pun)

Obviously we can all wear nearly any colour we want. But it is the undertone of our skin that determines which colours look best on us. Before we move on, let me just explain some of the science at work here. You might remember some of this from your art classes at school.

All colours have three main characteristics: Undertone, Clarity & Depth.

All colours contain yellow and blue. Colours can be categorised as either **warm,** which means they have a **yellow** undertone and this just means the colour has more yellow in it than blue. Or **cool,** which means they have a **blue** undertone meaning the colour has more blue in it than yellow.

As our skin, hair and eyes react to the colours around them, the first step in selecting your best colours is to match the warmth or coolness of the colours to your personal undertone.

Then we decide the clarity of the colour based on how bright or muted it is. For example a lime green is warm and bright and a moss green is warm and muted. Finally the depth of the colour is either deep or light, navy blue being cool and deep and powder blue being cool and light. Stylists measure the depth on a scale of 1 – 10. 1 being black and 10 being white. Can you imagine all the different shades there are in between?

We are now going to explore colour undertone, clarity and depth. This section is about finding what colours are more suited to your undertone.

STYLISH

Finding your undertone ...

So let's begin by finding out if you are a **yellow** or a **blue** undertone

Make sure your face is free of make up and your hair is pulled back off your face. Use a band if your hair is dyed to get a better analysis. If you have been on a sun bed or use any kind of tanning products you will have to concentrate closely on your eyes.

You'll need the colour cards from the style kit in your Box of Secrets, so when you have them, sit in front of the mirror at the window in natural daylight. Now I know that you probably don't like any of the colours on them but that's not the point, I want you to get a really clear and exaggerated picture of colour here, I know you'd probably never wear any of these but the shades have been specifically chosen to make it really easy for you to see the effect that colour has on your skin.

Ok, let's begin, Make sure you are completely make up free so you can concentrate on what the colours are doing to your face. Remove your top garment (sorry for being so forward especially as we've not met yet) and make sure no other colours can be seen around your face. Each colour will affect how your face looks, sometimes quite dramatically. Please do not look at the colour at all. Concentrate on your face.

Take each card in turn and place it underneath your neck just resting on the collar bone. At first, just try them all, one after another and get a feel for which card you instinctively prefer. I can't stress this enough, not which colour you prefer but which version of your face you prefer.

Are your eyes brighter, is that spot or blemish more noticeable and is your overall appearance much clearer and even? Notice that if you have a spot or blemish, placing a colour that has the correct undertone for your skin next to your face will calm the redness but if the colour is wrong for your undertone it will make the spots look redder and more obvious.

Now – go through the colours again one at a time, hold them under your chin resting on your collar bone and focus on the area under your eyes. Is it darker or lighter with the different colours, do you look tired and drawn or bright and glowing? Another common area to notice any difference is underneath your neck. Some colours will add light and some add shade giving the illusion of a wider or thinner appearance to the neck. Just concentrate on these areas of the face and neck for now as you try the different cards.

You are your own best judge for this and only you know what you want to enhance and what you want to hide. Remember the colour that suits will make the whites of your eyes whiter and your appearance fresher. The colours that don't will add shadows under the eyes and increase the appearance of blemishes. You can do this as often as you like till you're happy with your choice.

Ok, so here's where it gets interesting, you now have your preferred option, just notice which one it is. We're going to just double check your preference against your hair and eye colour next.

Warm Bright – Bright green
Warm Muted – Olive green
Cool Bright – Fuchsia
Cool Muted – Powder Pink

Warm and Bright – Bright Green brought out the best in you
Characteristically your hair will be golden blonde, strawberry blonde, strawberry red, auburn, golden brown, red or sandy grey.

Your skin will look ivory, ivory with golden freckles, peach, golden beige or rosy cheeks.

Your eyes will be blue, clear blue, clear green, turquoise, bright blue or light golden brown.

You will suit bright green, coral, salmon, peach, light gold, clear bright aqua, clear bright pink, blue violet, mango and turquoise.

Warm and Muted – Olive Green brought out the best in you
Characteristically your hair will be red, copper, chestnut, golden brown, charcoal black (red highlights) or golden grey.

Your skin will be ivory with golden freckles, golden beige, peach with golden freckles, dark coppery beige or black with a golden undertone.

Your eyes will be dark brown, golden brown, amber, hazel, green or blue with turquoise.

You will suit oyster, mustard, gold, dark chocolate brown, olive green, autumn grey, dark tomato red, dark teal, marine navy, warm purple, forest green.

Cool and Bright – Fuchsia brought out the best in you
Characteristically your hair will be blue black, medium brown (reddish highlight), dark brown (grey beige tone), salt and pepper, silver grey, white blonde or silver white.

Your skin will be very white (lily), white with pink undertone, beige (can be sallow), rose beige, olive, black with a blue undertone and charcoal freckles.

Your eyes will be brown, hazel, grey blue, blue, dark blue, grey green or green.

You will suit dark true red, chinese blue, bright lemon yellow, deep hot pink, emerald green, navy blue, aubergine, charcoal grey, royal purple, fuschia and black.

Cool and Muted – Powder Pink brought out the best in you
Characteristically your hair will be platinum blonde, ash blonde, blonde brown, light brown, brown grey (beige tone), brown with some auburn or blue grey.

Your skin colour will be peaches and cream, beige/lily with pink cheeks, beige/lily with no colour, rose coloured freckles or charcoal freckles.

Your eye colour will be cloudy blue with brown around the pupil, grey blue, grey green, pale grey, green, blue, hazel, bright blue or turquoise.

You will suit plum, lavender, sky blue, pastel pink, powder pink, light periwinkle blue, soft white, light lemon yellow, rose brown and deep blue green.

Which one brings out the best in you? I hope that by now you should fit comfortably into one of the undertones. If you're not quite there yet, just take the time to sit in front of your mirror at the window and look into your eyes. Write down all the colours you see. Then write down your natural hair colour and finally look at your skin. Have you got freckles or are your blue veins very obvious?

Below is a list of Neutral colours that you can base your wardrobe around depending on your undertone. Neutrals are the foundation of your wardrobe. You may have heard the phrase 'capsule wardrobe'

Normally this consists of 2 skirts, 2 pairs of trousers, one suit and 2 jackets. You can then build on that by adding blouses, t-shirts, jumpers and accessories and start dressing with ease every morning effortlessly.

Cool Undertone
Black and Grey
White
Navy
Taupe
Burgundy
Pine Green
Cherry Red

Warm Undertone
Brown
Rust
Cream
Camel
Teal
Olive
Tomato Red

If you are a Cool Undertone, why not have a little fun and buy a burgundy skirt for a change instead of black/navy and if you are a Warm Undertone try on that olive green jacket for the office instead of black/navy. You'll be surprised just how many people tell you how great you look. Too many women limit their clothes to black, grey, navy and white. Bring a little adventure into your wardrobe.

Shape

Face Section

Now you have all the colours sorted out, we are going to move straight onto face and then body shape. You can use your pull out for this. We will work from head to toe and start with your face shape first. Pull your hair away from your face and look into the mirror using your face shape tool. Hold it out comfortably and fit your face into one of the eight shapes. Make sure you can see the chin, jaw and forehead.

STYLISH

Oblong: The face is longer than it is wide with the cheek, jaw and forehead being of equal length.

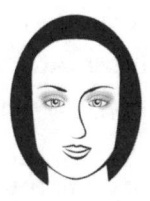

Stylists top tip
+ Go for short layered bobs. A fringe will reduce the length of the face. Hair parted off centre. Wispy styles onto the face.
  An ideal style of hair cut will create width at the sides and give the illusion of a wider face.
− Avoid long straight flat styles that will emphasize the long facial lines.

Oval: The face length is noticeably longer than the width. The forehead is slightly wider than the chin.

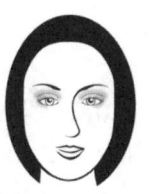

Stylists top tip
+ Considered the ideal face shape, most hairstyles will suit this face shape. Take hair condition and hairline into account though when choosing a style for yourself.
− Avoid centre partings and thick straight fringes as they will give the illusion of a wider forehead.

Round: The cheekbones are wider than the forehead and jaw line. Often has a round hairline and round jaw.

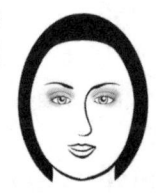

Stylists top tip
+ Add height to the top and shape onto the face reducing the width. Round face shapes lack the length of the oval face so hair should be cut to create the illusion of length in the face. Reduce hair width by keeping it flat at the sides and around the ears.
- Avoid centre partings, very short or full styles, round styles and tight curls, flat hair and very short hair that will emphasize the round face shape.

Square: The forehead, cheekbones and jaw line are similar width. The width is 2/3 or more of the length.

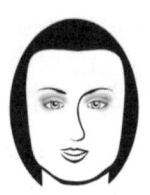

Stylists top tip
+ Adding height to the crown will give the illusion of a longer face. Use layers to create movement at the temples and sides as this will soften bone structure. Create wisps around the face to reduce squareness.
- Avoid chin length bobs as they will make your face look short and wide. Thick straight cut fringes will shorten the length of the face.

Inverted Triangular or Heart shaped: Has a wide forehead and narrowness across the jaw line.

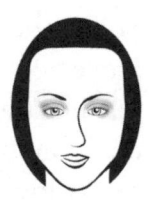

Stylists top tip
+   A flicked out bob would be good, adding volume or waves at the jaw line to help create fullness across the chin. Fringes are good to reduce the breadth of the forehead.
−   Avoid styles that are pulled back off the forehead and thick straight fringes that will add width to the forehead. Adding too much height may portray the narrowness of the chin and mouth.

Diamond: Cheekbones are wider than the forehead and jaw line. The jaw line is angular and pointed.

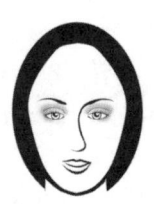

Stylists top tip
+   Flicked out bobs will suit this shape to help create fullness at the jaw line. Keep the hair close to the face with fullness across the forehead. A short style with fullness at the temples and brushed back across the ears. By creating width at the forehead and minimising it at the cheekbones you will give the illusion of an oval face.
−   Avoid centre partings and styles that will add volume at the cheekbone. Flat hair at the temples will emphasize the face length.

Stylists bonus top tip for colouring your hair …

Have you ever thought about getting your hair coloured but just didn't know where to start? It is a very difficult decision to make as your hair can make all the difference to the look you want to create. So here are a few tips.

- Always ask a professional before colouring your hair if you have never had it coloured before. There are chemicals in most hair colourings that can cause a reaction so it is always better to seek professional advice.
- Have a good think about the look you want to create.
- Do not go too dark or too light too soon as this might scare you into dying it again to dull it down or brighten it, then it can all go wrong.
- Tell your stylist your undertone.

Cool undertones will suit ashy shades of brown rather than red-browns.

Warm undertones will suit golden, rich brown and redder colourings.

And … Relax …

There's a lot to take in, so how are you getting on? Don't get too hung up on 'I can't do this, I don't get it, this isn't working.'

I would like you now to go back to the colour process and read it again. Sit down and relax and really think about it. Look at yourself in the mirror again. Look at how many colours you have in your eyes. Yes, I bet they are gorgeous. Look at the shape of your eyebrows, nose, chin, jaw, forehead. Really look at yourself intimately for the first time. You are an amazing woman and you should celebrate this. Now, go back to the face shapes and try again even if you think you got it right first time.

Many women (and men for that matter) beat themselves up too easily. We all complain about one thing or another and do you know what? It doesn't matter. It may also be because everybody else is doing it. People in the office, at home, in the playground, in the supermarket. It's a habit of complaining and wishing things were different. I have worked with some very, very beautiful women, top models, actresses and beauty queens and I'll tell you that every one of them has something that they don't like about their body or face or hair. Why should it be any different for you? But you can do something about it now, this is the time to stop wishing and grab some of the secrets that the stars use to make yourself feel better about being you.

So be different. Instead of just wishing you were richer, happier, prettier, slimmer … … go get it all. This whole process will assist you in doing that, so well done you for getting this far.

We are going to move comfortably onto body shapes. I know what you're thinking but I would like you to imagine your body as a new project.

Let go of your own vision of yourself and place yourself as your very own personalised Image Consultant.

I want you to find an area where you can comfortably undress and look at yourself in the mirror. A full length mirror is recommended. If you have not got one at home, go to any clothes shop and hide in a cubicle.

Body shape section

Assessing your own body shape

Our body shapes are pre-determined genetically and are largely dependent on bone size and fat allocation. Women can have either a bowl shaped pelvis which is typical of the female curves or a male shaped pelvis which is typical of straighter bottom half and well shaped legs.

Every woman has an area of her body she dislikes or wants to change. It may be a flabby tummy or underarms, big tummy or small breasts. So you're not alone when you think 's**t, they want me to look at myself naked in the mirror'. Sorry but I really do. It's our little secret remember ... but being completely honest and knowing what to look for in yourself is the only place to begin. This is about really getting to know your own shape and learning how to work with your body to enhance your natural assets. There are lots of ways to hide and enhance our shapes but I'm told that the best place to start is in the underwear department.

Stylists top tip
A well fitted bra will transform any outfit as well as completely change the way you look. It may also alter the size of clothes you buy too.

Ok, I know I'm labouring the point now but this next exercise works best if you are standing in front of a full length mirror naked. This way you can fully see all areas.

Start from the face and work your way down asking yourself these questions. Just jot your answers down here …

Are my shoulders Straight – Curvy – Narrow – Broad?
Is my back Narrow – Broad?
Are my breasts Small, Medium or Large?
Do I have a waist?
Is my bottom Round or Flat?
Are my hips Straight or Curved?
Are my calves Straight or Curved?

Have a read through the following body shapes before deciding which is most like you.

Figure of 8 is the body shape most women aspire to have. Curved shoulders, full bust, noticeable waist and curved hips and thighs. You will find all waistbands are loose on you. Hipsters are a good choice. You will feel more comfortable in soft flowing fabrics that have added lycra, soft wools and knits, light suede, fine corduroy and soft linen and silk.

There can be two versions of the figure of 8, slim and petite or fuller and curvy.

Fabric needs to be soft.

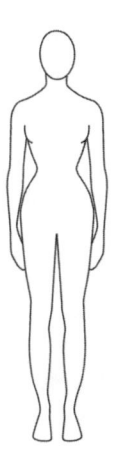

Stylists top tip
The aim is to accentuate a small waist and a feminine shape, avoiding a box look. If a straight style is chosen the fabric has to be soft and have added lycra.

Clothing lines:

Jackets	– shaped to enhance the waist, curved lapels, shawl collar, minimal detail at the bust. Single breasted, straight open cardigans.
Skirts	– side button or zip, wrap over, adjustable waistband, bias cut.
Trousers	– hipsters, side button or zip, minimal detail e.g. no pockets.
Tops	– wrap over, curved neckline, twinsets and shaped in soft fabric.
Dresses	– wrap overs, shaped, bias cut, swing bottom all in soft fabrics with added lycra.

Avoid crisp cotton fabric as this will not follow your natural body lines and may give you a boxy look, hiding your waist. The aim is to create a natural balance without adding bulk.

Oval is curved at the shoulders and back, your middle is fuller than your bust. Well shaped legs.

Stylists top tip
Choose soft flowing fabrics with straight lines to avoid the illusion of bulkiness. Fabrics such as light to medium weight e.g. smooth wools and knits, chiffon, light suede, velvet, taffeta, linen, silk.

Emphasise the shoulder line and keep attention on the face.

Choose loose fitting longer line tops, without drawing attention to the waist. Soft gathers or elasticated waists are best.

Clothing lines:
Jackets – unstructured, long straight styles, cardigans long and straight, no collar.
Skirts – bias cut, wrap, elasticated.
Trousers – softer culottes, elasticated, simple.
Tops – necklines to flatter bust, shoulder pads, loose fitted long blouses, simple.
Dresses – A-line, bias cut, swagger

Avoid anything too fitted, too short, too detailed, t-shirts unless loose, any fabric that clings.

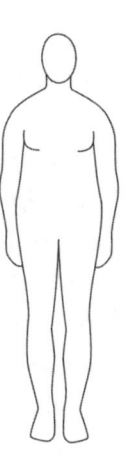

Pear shape has narrow curved shoulders, noticeable waist, full hips and thighs.

Stylists top tip
You will feel more comfortable in soft flowing materials with minimal patterns on your bottom half while your top half can afford to have lots of detail e.g. pockets, patterns, buttons and layers.

Fabrics light to medium weight. Cotton, linen, wool, suede and corduroy. Hipsters are a good choice for trousers. Create the illusion that your top half is balanced with your bottom half by using layers, patterns and detail on the top.

Clothing lines:

Jackets	– double breasted, detailed, pockets and buttons, shoulder pads
Skirts	– flat fronted, softly pleated, wrap, bias cut, side button or zip
Trousers	– hipsters, flat fronted, side button or zip.
Tops	– shaped to emphasise the waist, twin sets, curved necklines, patterns, dots and weaves
Dresses	– you may find it difficult to get your size as the top half is smaller than the bottom half. Tailor made or two piece would be a better choice.

Avoid short skirts and too much detail on the bottom half. Keep all the detail and attention on the top half.

Inverted Triangle has wide straight shoulders with narrower hips. There is no noticeable difference between the waist and hips.

Stylists top tip
Keep the designs simple and use colour instead of patterns.

Avoid shoulder pads or anything which makes your shoulders appear wider than they really are. Remember it's all about perspective and you want to give the illusion of perfect proportions.

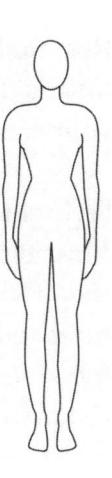

Clothing lines:
Jackets   – simple design, slightly fitted, peplum, boxy, bolero, chanel, bomber.
Skirts   – short skirts, straight, pleated, panelled.
Trousers – suits all, add detail to accentuate bottom.
Tops   – v-neck, straight, simple, halter
Dresses   – simple, shaped, shift

THE SLIM GIRL'S BOOK OF SECRETS

Rectangle: Your silhouette is almost straight up and down. There is little difference between your waist and hips.

Stylists top tip
Most clothes can be worn well on this body shape but the cut of cloth needs to be structured with a strong shoulder line. The lean figure can add layers and the fuller figure should avoid drawing attention to a wide waist. Aim to create a shape.

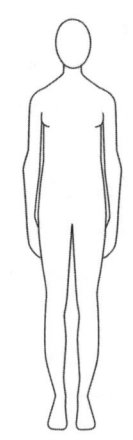

Clothing lines:

Jackets	– shaped, single or double breasted, long semi fitted cardigans
Skirts	– straight, pencil, straight wrap, panelled, side or front buttons and zips
Trousers	– go for anything you like as you can wear almost every design
Tops	– v-neck, straight, simple, halter, tank, straight lapels
Dresses	– simple, straight, shift, halter

If this is you, you're a lucky thing this body shape can wear almost anything and look great.

Keyhole: Straight shoulder line can have a full back, noticeable waist, full thighs and hips. Emphasise the small waist.

Stylists top tip
Top half of the body suits a more structured clothing line and the curves on the bottom half need something a bit softer with added lycra.

Avoid shoulder pads and stiff fabric on the lower half of the body.

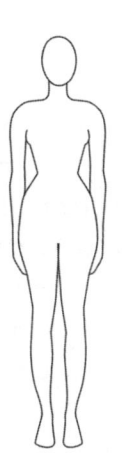

Clothing lines:
Jackets	– simple design, slightly fitted, peplum, boxy, bolero, chanel, bomber
Skirts	– side button or zip, wrap over, adjustable waistband, bias cut
Trousers	– hipsters, side button or zip, minimal detail e.g. no pockets
Tops	– v-neck, straight, simple, halter
Dresses	– v-neck, added lycra, bias, simple

Dress to your own scale and proportion i.e. small, medium or large boned. This means keeping the size of your accessories, patterns, heels on shoes etc to the same scale. Imagine putting Dawn French in a pair of kitten heels or Kylie Minogue in a clumpy heel. Create a balance which will be pleasing to the eye.

> '*Fashion fades, style lingers*'
> *Yves St Laurent*

Style is not just about clothes. Consider your lifestyle, personality and budget. Think about how you live your life. What does your style say about you?

The fashion industry cannot cater for every woman on the planet so it's good to know what to look out for yourself. The new look this season may not be your style and you will look and feel uncomfortable if you buy something that's just not you. Shopping should be fun.

You will save money and time when you know what suits you.

Remember this? You are going to an event where you need a special outfit. You buy an expensive dress. It cost £150 and looked amazing on the hanger and in the advert. You put it on ready for the big night and feel deflated because it's not as nice on you as the picture you had in your mind so, you wear it once then it goes to the back of the wardrobe.

Or, you buy a wonderful outfit because you know it's your style and colour and you will wear it again. Wear it 10 times and it has cost you £15 per wear. I want you to really get into the habit of working out the likely Cost Per Wear (CPW) of an outfit before you buy it. It is so important to build your wardrobe and really make it work for you. How many items do you have in your wardrobe that you never wear? You can rescue them by using accessories such as scarves and jewellery.

There are a few simple guidelines you can follow when buying an outfit to help you along the way. But remember before you buy anything work out the CPW.

Imagine wrapping 2 items. One is a ball, the other is a box of chocolates. You would probably use soft paper for the ball and something a bit stiffer for the chocolates. The same thing applies to dressing your body using fabrics.

There are many reasons why we all don't fit into the standard sizes of many stores. Do you sometimes find you are a size smaller or bigger depending on what store you go into? The most common reason is because we are all different body shapes. And so different styles and fabrics will look very different on different people. The good news is we are going to help you assess your own body shape and dress it to its full potential.

Stylists Top Tip

Choose the correct fabric
Have you ever considered fabric when buying an item of clothing? Have you ever put on an outfit then spent the whole day fidgeting with your bra straps or unbuttoning your skirt or trousers, had to take that jacket or cardigan off as soon as you get to work? Chances are it's a style or fabric that just doesn't work for you. It's not your fault and not a problem, there are more than enough styles out there, but … you might need to loosen the image you have of yourself and try something new for a change.

Stylists Top Tip

Never allow anything to finish at your widest point. For example if you have wide hips, buying a jacket that stops at your widest point will only accentuate your wide hips. If you have large calves, buying a skirt that stops on the widest point of your calves will only attract the eye to that area.

Enhancing and minimising guidelines.
Do's and Don'ts.

Long neck.
+ Do wear polo necks and turtle necks, chokers and scarves.
− Don't wear low v-necks, very long, narrow earrings.

Short necks.
+ Do wear v-necks, low neckline, open collars, longer necklaces.
− Don't wear high necklines, scarves or chokers.

Large bust.
+ Do wear a well fitted bra, v-necks, non clinging fabric, darker colours, vertical lines, minimal fuss.
− Don't wear high necklines, plain fronted t-shirts, puffed sleeves, jewellery falling onto the bust, breast pockets, wide belts, horizontal lines.

Small bust.
+ Do wear layers, detail, pockets across bust line, horizontal lines, lighter colours, plain t-shirts, t-shirt bra.
− Don't wear tight fitting garments, clinging fabrics or low cut tops.

Noticeable tummy area.
+ Do wear flat fronted skirts and trousers, side buttons and zips, good underwear, darker colours, blouson tops.
− Don't wear short tops including jackets, wide belts, front detail, anything tight.

Fuller thighs & hips.
+ Do wear shoulder pads to create a balance, darker colours on the bottom half of the body, vertical designs, good underwear, straight styles. Jackets and tops that fall below or above the widest point.
− Don't wear short skirts, pockets, light shiny fabrics, horizontal designs, leggings, clingy fabric.

What's in your wardrobe?

Below is an example of how one woman spends her week and we compare it to her wardrobe,

Monday: work, lunch with friends, aerobics in the evening
Tuesday: work, meetings, out for drinks in the evening
Wednesday: work, then straight home
Thursday: work, then straight home
Friday: work, out for dinner and drinks

Saturday: catch up with housework, shopping, then cinema in the evening
Sunday: family round for roast dinner

Her wardrobe may look something like this:

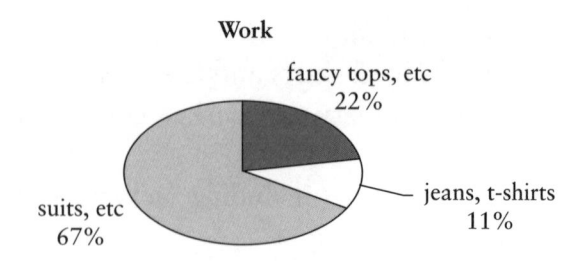

Work

- fancy tops, etc 22%
- jeans, t-shirts 11%
- suits, etc 67%

Because she is at work most of the week, her wardrobe has a large percentage of work clothes, like suits and shirts, and socialising clothes, like evening tops with dressy trousers next and gym outfits, etc. make up a smaller percentage.

Draw one of your own charts, then have a look in your wardrobe and decide what you need to change. Try and save as much money as you can by accessorizing your t-shirts, for example, by adding a necklace or earrings or a brooch.

Wardrobe Workout

Your mission now is to rescue as much as possible. Make three piles of clothes. This is great fun and may surprise you – it certainly did me.

Pile 1 Items you only wear once a year (special occasions, holiday, swimwear, etc.)
Pile 2 Items you haven't worn for more than 6 months
Pile 3 All your other clothes

Once a Year Pile
Start with those items that you only wear once a year and decide if you will definitely need them again this year. If not, put them outside the door. This will become your charity or swap pile. If you will wear them again, really? Will you? Put them back in the wardrobe.

Not Worn for over 6 Months
This pile you will probably never wear again. Here are a few reasons you may have or excuses for still having them in your wardrobe.

1. Impulsive buy – the price tag might even still be on it?
2. Don't know why but you just don't like it – who cares it's time to say good bye!
3. Lost weight – there will be quite a few of these, all evidence of your success.
4. It's not comfortable – this could be because it's the wrong cut or fabric for you. What's the point of keeping something that doesn't make you feel great?
5. It cost me a lot of money – and it's spent. You can't take clothes to the bank or pay the gas bill with a cheeky little blouse. It's too late for this one but the

secrets you've gained here will ensure you don't make the same mistake again.
6. I bought it because it was in the sale – ah, my favourite but it's only a bargain (even on sale) if it has a low CPW.

Ring any bells for you?

Assess if you can rescue any of these items by accessorizing or wearing with something else. If you won't wear them again put them on the charity pile.

All Other Clothes

Go through this pile slowly, checking fabric and general condition of the item. Are there any buttons missing? Is it stained? Does it need to be dry cleaned? If so, create a 'to be fixed' pile and take action to resurrect those items (it's cheaper than buying new ones) Then put the rest back into your wardrobe and drawers. Change the drawers around to give that new feeling to the exercise.

Hang all your jackets next to each other, then all your skirts and repeat this with trousers, blouses, jumpers, etc. Eventually you will be able to go into your wardrobe and pick an outfit with ease and when they are all in your colours you can mix and match your suits and shirts and skirts to create numerous wonderful outfits.

Stylists top tip
It is well worth investing in good wooden hangers or thick plastic ones. The thin wired ones can ruin your clothes.

All the clothes that are outside your door need to be bagged as soon as possible. This is important as you'll probably feel the need to go through them again and you will be using your emotional attachments to keep something you have just decided to give away.

You should now feel invigorated as if you have just had a real workout. Well done you!

Make up – the finishing touch.

Finally, I am going to take you through a makeup workout which will put the icing on the cake of the new you. This will guide you through some beauty secrets of the stars. Follow these few steps to create a fresh natural complexion and all you will need to do is add more colour for a night out or special occasion. Apply in order after you have cleansed, toned and moisturised.

Concealer is excellent for brightening up dark circles underneath the eye. Pat gently with your finger.

Stylists Top Tip
+ Yellow concealer helps counteract dark circles under the eye.
+ Blue concealer is used to neutralise tan spots and is great for age spots and dark freckles.
+ Green concealer is used to counteract redness or blemishes or scars.
+ Lavender concealer is used to neutralise unwanted yellow tones.

+ Light Mauve concealer helps to counteract bruises and facial veins.

Foundation is used to create a flawless look and a blank canvas. The colour should be slightly darker than your undertone. If it's an exact match it may pale you. Dab on where needed and use a foundation brush to blend. When choosing a colour it is best to go for 3 you think are close to your skin shade, then dab a sample of each on your forehead in line with each other. Go for the one that blends the best without being too light or too dark.

Powder. Apply loosely in your shade using a powder puff or brush

Blusher. Apply blusher by smiling and brush up onto the apples of the cheeks. Brush downwards to blend.

Lipstick or gloss.
By now you will be very familiar with whether you suit cool shades or warm shades and which colours really work for you. Here's a quick guide to which shades of lipstick will work for you.

Cool shades. Plum, fuchsia, raspberry, rose pink, burgundy, red
Warm shades. Gold, coral, bronze, copper, cinnabar, tomato red

Lip Liner Pencil.
If your lips are thin, apply pencil on the outside of the lip line.

If your lips are full, apply on the inside of the lip line.
If you love your lips, apply on the lip line.
Tip – Try and use the same shade as lipstick or gloss.

Eye shadow.
Apply a light colour from lash to brow as a base. Your eye shape will determine how you apply colour.

The Eyes have it

Close set eyes
Apply lighter shades towards the inside of the eye and start to blend darker shades outwards. Use eye liner pencil from the middle of the eyelid to outward corners. Repeat on bottom outside lid, middle to outwards to join upper line

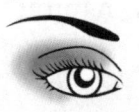

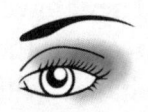

Almond eyes
Considered to be the perfect eye shape, so you can have some fun using different techniques. You will suit them all.

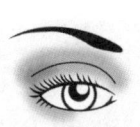

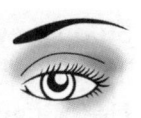

Protruding Bulging eyes
Use medium shade all over the eye from lash to brow. Add a darker shade from lash to socket. Use liner on top and bottom and lots of mascara. Wow!

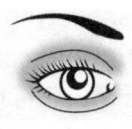

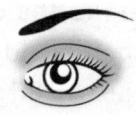

Hooded eyes

This normally happens as we get older. The skin loses some of its elasticity and we end up with what seems to be a fold in the socket. Don't worry, using medium to darker shades will bring your eyes back to life. Try using really light shades just near the inner corner to brighten the eye.

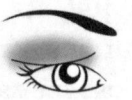

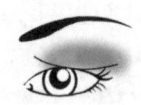

Deep Set eyes

They have a natural shadow around them so using lighter shades will bring the eyes out more. Use a light base all over including just under the bottom lashes, then enhance with a light medium under the socket and blend up and out going no further than the eyebrow. This eye shape works well with sparkly shadow. Go and buy it now for your next night out.

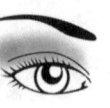

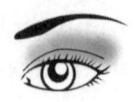

Sloping eyes

The aim here is to lift the eye. Use a light base all over, then add a darker shade halfway along the eye socket and work outwards. Blend, blend then blend again to create the smoky effect. Use liner on the top lid from outside the eye bringing it halfway along and keeping it as close to the lashes as you can.

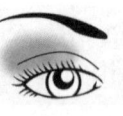

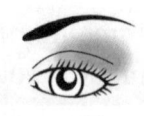

Eye liner. Line the upper lash area with an eye shadow colour applied with a eye liner brush. This gives a softer look or use a pencil to be a bit more dramatic. If applying liner to the bottom lid make sure it's even with the top and meets at the corner of the outer eye.

Mascara. If you are a warm undertone use brown/black and cool go for black, keep it simple but don't be afraid of a little change.

Style journal
My natural hair colour is _____
My natural skin colour is _____
My face shape is _____
My body shape is _____
My favourite colour for me is _____
The most daring colour for me is _____
The best fabric for me is _____
My favourite part of me is my _____
The part I don't beat myself up about any more is my
_____

Conclusion

Thank you so much for taking the time to allow me to help. It has been my pleasure to sit and write this short, but hopefully fun, guide to living a slimmer, fitter, healthier and more active life. It's been a lot of fun and I hope you've enjoyed it too.

There are 2 things you can do now, you can either pop this book back in the box and stick it on the shelf beside all your others, but, that won't achieve very much …

Or, you can use this as the starting point for a journey that will take you to new and exciting places. It never fails to amaze me just how quickly or to what extent peoples' lives can change for the better once they start doing things, even just a little bit differently.

I know people who now live the life they once only dreamed of just by making a few simple changes in their lives. It really can be very simple. I have seen people use just some of the techniques in this book to earn more money, improve their relationships, eliminate illness, stress and pain, and, of course, lose lots of weight in the process. You have in your hands some of the very best techniques I have used over the years with people the world over.

Weight loss is not the dark art that the diet industry would have you believe, the biggest secret is that there is no secret to losing weight except using what you have here and getting on and doing it.

I don't know which section has been your favourite or which will have the greatest impact on your life but I do know that if you use what you've learned, there can only be one outcome. You will almost inevitably change your life for the better. I'd like you to think of this as the beginning of something rather than the end of a book.

My coaching style is to try to help my clients in any way I can and you are no different. My goal is to help you on your journey and I would love to share your success with you. My take on coaching can best be summed up in the following text from the Chicago Tribune.

In the Olympics of Life, We Could All Use a Coach

by Mary Schmich; Chicago Tribune; February 18, 1998

I want a coach. Not a coach as in Cinderella's renovated pumpkin. Not a Coach as in a pricey shoulder bag. I want a coach like an Olympic coach. I want a coach to tune me up and calm me down, a coach to sigh for me and cry for me, a coach who'll rev me up to be all that I can be and take half the blame when I wind up bumbling through the triple lutz of life.

I want a coach like Picabo Street's coach, a coach who when Street had an injured knee and wanted to scope out the Olympic course skied her down the mountain on his back. I want a coach who picks me up when I hurt, the way Bela Karolyi carried gymnast Kerri Strug and her injured ankle to collect her summer gold. I want a coach like all those rapt, devoted coaches I see perched on the Olympic sidelines in Nagano this winter, their faces turned toward their little darlings like sunbathers basking in the sun.

I want a coach who when I win envelopes me in hugs. I want a coach who when I lose envelopes me in hugs. I want a coach who when I've given all I've got wipes my brow and brings me cans of Coke. I want a coach to help me give it all I've got.

I want a coach – a life coach. I want someone whose life work is to better me, me, me, whose grand dreams are for me, me, me, who lives vicariously through moi!

A mere personal trainer will not do. Neither will a teacher. And a therapist? Gold cannot be won through talk. My life coach will be a personal trainer, a teacher, and a therapist all rolled into one, someone whose prime goal on this planet is to teach me tricks of mind and muscle, someone who'll show me how to leap and stretch and play through pain, someone who'll water the fields of my possibilities with expectation, consolation, congratulation and faith.

My life coach will see promise where others see a drearily blank slate. My life coach will invest in me as if I'm a hot new stock. My life coach will drill into my unrealized potential and extract a pot of gold.

My life coach will be a parent, only better. My coach will understand I own the power. My coach will not be distracted by household chores. My coach will be a parent who never makes me waste my talent scrubbing toilets.

I'd be a contender if I had a coach. Wouldn't you? Who wouldn't be a thousand times better, in everything from tooth brushing to planning out a life, if they had a coach to show them how it should be done, how much better it could be done, how much there is to win when it's done right?

Who would all those Olympic athletes be without a coach? They'd be the rest of us. Ok, maybe not that bad, but then again, not as good. Watch the Olympic coaches in Nagano, watch the way they watch their protégés. Don't you want a dose of that attention? Don't you want a life coach?

Most of us are slipping and sliding on the bumpy ice of life. Our execution's sloppy; we are poorly trained. We need some undistracted steering and grooming, prodding and propping up. We need someone to persuade us when we fail to get back on the ice, the slope, the course. All of us could benefit from someone who is always there to beam good wishes from the sidelines.

Instead, most of us slog through on our own, schlepping our untapped potential like unpacked suitcases waiting for a key. We get help from friends, lovers, spouses, mentors, parents, teachers, therapists, personal trainers, priests, rabbis, and TV talk-show hosts. But most of them have a limited attention span. None is devoted just to us. Most of them are just like us, feeling underused and unsung. They, too, are wishing for a coach. Think how spectacular it could be – the putty that is you placed in the hands of the right coach. Your coach, like a potter, would find the work of art straining to escape the clay.

There are loathsome coaches, sure. There are coaches who are dictators and Svengalis and ordinary louts. Not my coach. My coach would carry me piggyback down a mountain and thank me afterward.

And Finally …

As I have said earlier the difference between success and failure is not difficult, it's simply the difference between doing it and not doing it and having some good guidance along the way. Success is not a destination, it's a journey and to help you on your journey I have built the Slim Girl's Box of Secrets online. Here you will find even more tips, tricks and techniques to help you on your way. You will find videos to watch, interviews with world leading experts and celebrities and web-casts where I will personally coach, support and guide you.

My aim is to give you as much support as you'll ever need and the web site is really where that'll happen. You will be able to make new friends with other slim girls and find people with the same interests and questions. You really are part of something now and we're going to look after you. Log on to **www.slimgirlsboxofsecrets.com,** set up your profile and have a browse around.

But, before I sign off from here, I'd like to leave you with a thought …

It doesn't matter what life throws at you … It's not worth being fat and miserable for! Live life on your terms and enjoy it, it's the only one you have for now …

Have fun! – Ali

Daily Do's

THE SLIM GIRL'S BOOK OF SECRETS

Day 1. Daily Do – Make a decision based purely on the flip of a coin.

Reflection – How long did you 'just sit' for?

My free space

___

Day 2. Daily Do – Pay someone a compliment – It's free!

Reflection – How many glasses of water did you drink today?

My free space

___

Day 3. Daily Do – Actively use different words. Don't get angry, get irked!

Reflection – How did you feel emotionally 1–10?

My free space

DAILY DO'S

Day 4. Daily Do – Enjoy it – Whatever you're doing.

Reflection – The thing I did to make my heart sing was?

My free space
___

Day 5. Daily Do – Just quit – just for the day.

Reflection – The best thing about today was?

My free space
___

Day 6. Daily Do – Allow yourself to just be.

Reflection – What did you stop trying to control?

My free space
___

Day 7. Daily Do – *Just sit.*

Reflection – Which struggle did you let go of?

My free space

Day 8. Daily Do – *Concentrate on the thing you most like about yourself.*

Reflection – How long did you 'just sit' for?

My free space

Day 9. Daily Do – *Do just one thing at a time and do it well.*

Reflection – How many glasses of water did you drink today?

My free space

DAILY DO'S

Day 10. Daily Do – Be flexible and allow yourself to flow.

Reflection – How did you feel emotionally 1–10?

My free space

Day 11. Daily Do – Make someone's day – Do something selfless for someone else.

Reflection – The thing I did to make my heart sing was?

My free space

Day 12. Daily Do – Do something that makes your heart sing. However small, just do a little thing that really makes you smile on the inside.

Reflection – The best thing about today was?

My free space

Day 13. Daily Do – Who would you like to have in your corner? Bring them into your life, even if it's just in your imagination.

Reflection – What did you stop trying to control?

My free space

Day 14. Daily Do – Trust your inner knowing – close your eyes, go inside, connect with your heart and ask. 'what do I need to do'? Trust your inner knowing.

Reflection – Which struggle did you let go of?

My free space

Day 15. Daily Do – You have only love at your core ... if you meet someone who is not aligned with you, send them love and move along.

Reflection – How long did you 'just sit' for?

My free space

DAILY DO'S

Day 16. Daily Do – Remember that people almost always act in the best way that they can given their circumstances. Cut people and yourself some slack.

Reflection – How many glasses of water did you drink today?

My free space

Day 17. Daily Do – Eat slowly

Reflection – How did you feel emotionally 1–10?

My free space

Day 18. Daily Do – Do little and often in everything you do.

Reflection – The thing I did to make my heart sing was?

My free space

Day 19. Daily Do – What's for you will not go by past you – unless you don't notice it. Open your eyes and your heart.

Reflection – The best thing about today was?

My free space

Day 20. Daily Do – You are emotional. Don't try to run your feelings with logic.

Reflection – What did you stop trying to control?

My free space

Day 21. Daily Do – There is no such thing as coincidence, notice what the universe is trying to tell you.

Reflection – Which struggle did you let go of?

My free space

DAILY DO'S

Day 22. Daily Do – You can do anything – If you have a good enough reason.

Reflection – How long did you 'just sit' for?

My free space

___

Day 23. Daily Do – Focus on what you DO want and attract it into your life.

Reflection – How many glasses of water did you drink today?

My free space

___

Day 24. Daily Do – Create a climate of wellbeing.

Reflection – How did you feel emotionally 1–10?

My free space

THE SLIM GIRL'S BOOK OF SECRETS

Day 25. Daily Do – Do you really want it? OR is it something you think you 'should' want.

Reflection – The thing I did to make my heart sing was?

My free space

Day 26. Daily Do – Let go and allow yourself to spring back to the real you.

Reflection – The best thing about today was?

My free space

Day 27. Daily Do – Listen to your gut instinct – it's usually right.

Reflection – What did you stop trying to control?

My free space

DAILY DO'S

Day 28. Daily Do – Follow your heart today and you'll last forever.

Reflection – Which struggle did you let go of?

My free space
___

Day 29. Daily Do – Set up a good feeling and anchor it.

Reflection – How long did you 'just sit' for?

My free space
___

Day 30. Daily Do – The Gardener's Guide to a Happy Day. Create the garden you want and 'attract' the things you want.

Reflection – How many glasses of water did you drink today?

My free space
___

*Day 31. Daily Do – **Stop repeating your story and start creating the next chapter.***

Reflection – How long did you 'just sit' for?

My free space

*Day 32. Daily Do – **Try a new look today, what do you dare to wear?***

Reflection – How many glasses of water did you drink today?

My free space

*Day 33. Daily Do – **Who would you like to be today? Live as if you have the essence of them inside of you.***

Reflection – How did you feel emotionally 1–10?

My free space

DAILY DO'S

Day 34. Daily Do – Enjoy it – Find a fun and creative way to burn a few extra calories today. What is it?

Reflection – The thing I did to make my heart sing was?

My free space

Day 35. Daily Do – Drink, Drink, Drink … how many glasses of water have you had today?

Reflection – The best thing about today was?

My free space